The Quick and Easy Anti-Inflammatory Delicacies

Simple Recipes to Restart your Metabolism

Thomas Jollif

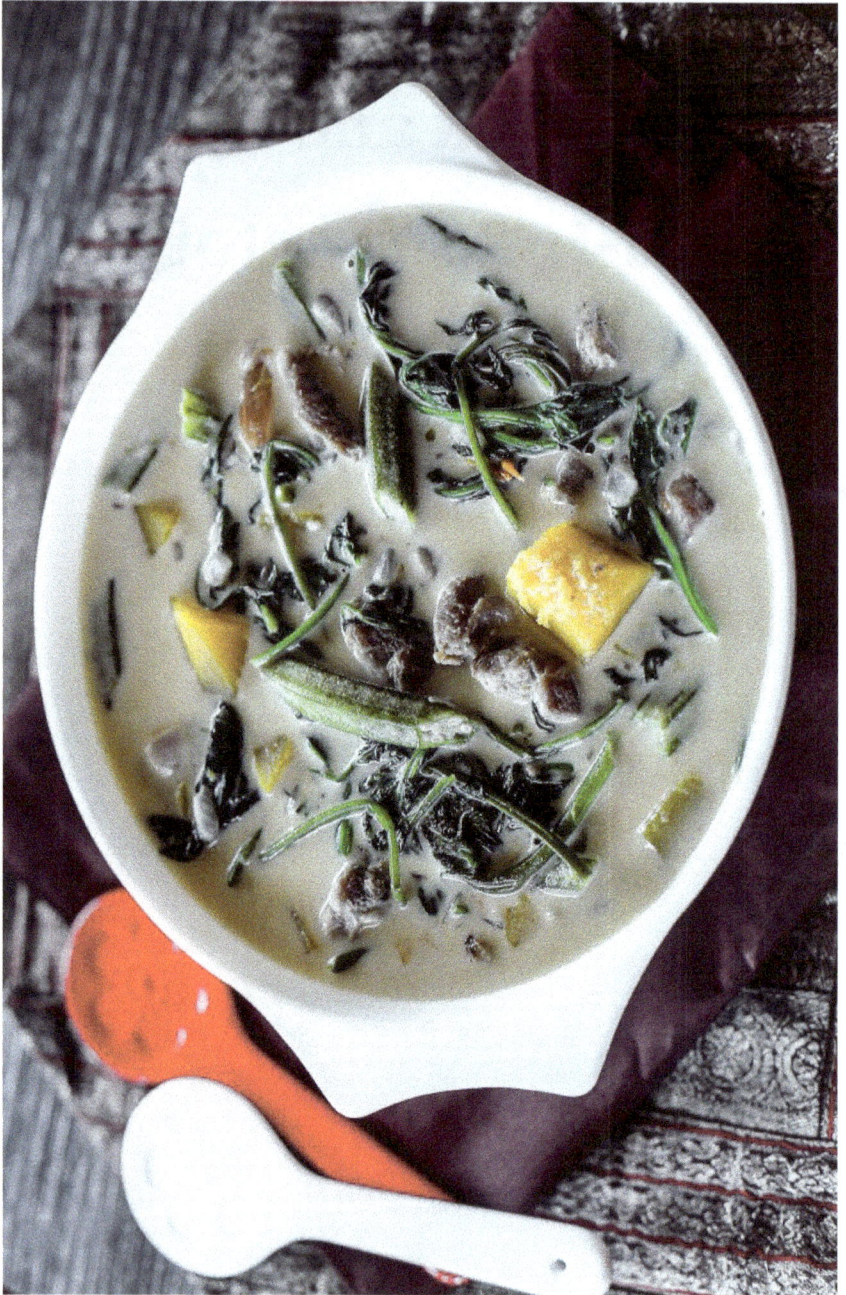

Table of Contents

BREAKFASTS

Kale Turmeric Scramble

Time To Prepare: five minutes

Time to Cook: ten minutes

Yield: Servings 1

Ingredients:

- ¼ tsp. Black pepper
- ½ cup Kale, shredded
- ½ cup Sprouts
- 1 tbsp. Garlic, minced
- 1 tbsp. Turmeric, ground
- 2 Eggs
- 2 tbsp. Olive oil

Directions:

1. Beat the eggs and put in in the turmeric, black pepper, and garlic. Sauté the kale into the olive oil on moderate heat for 5 minutes, and then pour this egg mixture into the pan with the kale.

2. Carry on cooking, frequently stirring, until the eggs are cooked to your preference. Top with raw sprouts before you serve.

Nutritional Info: Calories 137 ‖ 8.4 grams Fat ‖ 7.9 grams carbs ‖ 4.8 grams fiber ‖ 1.8grams sugar ‖ 13.2 grams protein

Leek & Spinach Frittata

Time To Prepare: ten minutes
Time to Cook: fifteen minutes
Yield: Servings 4

Ingredients:

- ½ Teaspoon Bail, Dried
- ½ Teaspoon Garlic Powder
- 1 Cup Baby Spinach, Fresh & Packed
- 1 Cup Cremini Mushrooms, Sliced
- 2 Leeks, Chopped Fine
- 2 Tablespoons Avocado Oil
- 8 Eggs
- Sea Salt & Black Pepper to Taste

Directions:

1. Set the oven to 400°F then get an ovenproof frying pan. Put it on moderate to high heat, sautéing your leeks in your avocado oil until tender. It should take roughly five minutes

2. Get out a container, and whisk the eggs with your garlic, basil, and salt. Put in them to the frying pan with your leeks, cooking for 5 minutes. You'll need to stir regularly.

3. Mix in your mushrooms and spinach, seasoning with pepper.

4. Put the frying pan in your oven then bake for about ten minutes. Serve warm.

Nutritional Info: Calories: 276 ‖ Protein: 19 Grams ‖ Fat: 17 Grams ‖ Carbohydrates: fifteen Grams

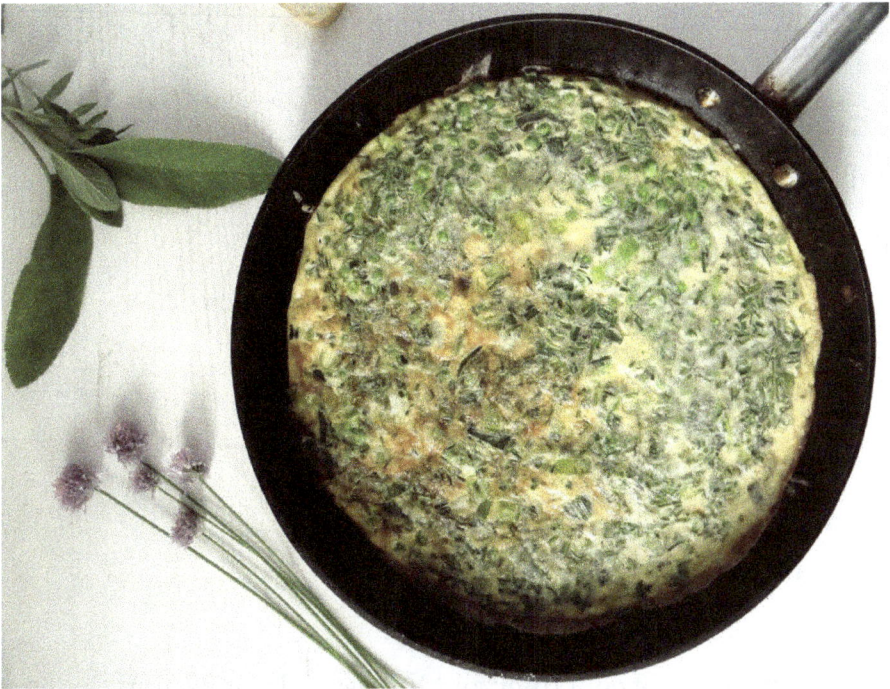

Mango Granola

Time To Prepare: ten minutes
Time to Cook: thirty minutes
Yield: Servings 4

Ingredients:

- ½ cup almonds, roughly chopped
- ½ cup dates, roughly chopped
- ½ cup nuts
- 1 cup dried mango, chopped
- 2 cups rolled oats
- 2 tbsp. coconut oil
- 2 tbsp. water
- 2 tsp. cinnamon
- 2/3 cup agave nectar
- 3 tbsp. sesame seeds

Directions:

1. Set oven at 320F
2. In a big container, put the oats, almonds, nuts, sesame seeds, dates, and cinnamon then mix thoroughly.

3. In the meantime, heat a deep cooking pan on moderate heat, pour in the agave syrup, coconut oil, and water.

4. Stir and allow it to cook for minimum 3 minutes or until the coconut oil has melted.

5. Slowly pour the syrup mixture into the container with the oats and nuts and stir thoroughly, make sure that all the ingredients are coated with the syrup.

6. Move the granola on a baking sheet coated with parchment paper and place in your oven to bake for about twenty minutes.

7. After twenty minutes, take off the tray from the oven and lay the chopped dried mango on top. Put back in your oven then bake again for another five minutes.

8. Allow the granola cool completely before you serve or placing it in an airtight container for storage. The shelf life of the granola will last up to 2-3 weeks.

Nutritional Info: Calories: 434 kcal ‖ Protein: 13.16 g ‖ Fat: 28.3 g ‖ Carbohydrates: 55.19 g

Maple Oatmeal

Time To Prepare: five minutes

Time to Cook: twenty minutes

Yield: Servings 4

Ingredients:

- ¼ cup Coconut flakes, unsweetened
- ½ cup Milk, almond or coconut
- ½ cup Pecans, chopped
- ½ cup Walnuts, chopped
- 1 tsp. Cinnamon
- 1 tsp. Maple flavoring
- 3 tbsp. Sunflower seeds
- 4 tbsp. Chia seeds

Directions:

1. Pulse the sunflower seeds, walnuts, and pecans in a food processor to crumble. Or you can just put the nuts in a sturdy plastic bag, wrap the bag using a towel, lay it on a sturdy surface, and beat the towel with a hammer until the nuts are crumbled.

2. Combine the crushed nuts with the remaining ingredients and pour them into a big pot. Simmer this mixture using low heat for thirty minutes. Stir

frequently, so the mix does not cling to the bottom. Serve decorated with fresh fruit or a drizzle of cinnamon if you wish.

Nutritional Info: Calories 374 ‖ 3.2 grams carbs ‖ 9.25 grams Protein ‖ 34.59 grams fat

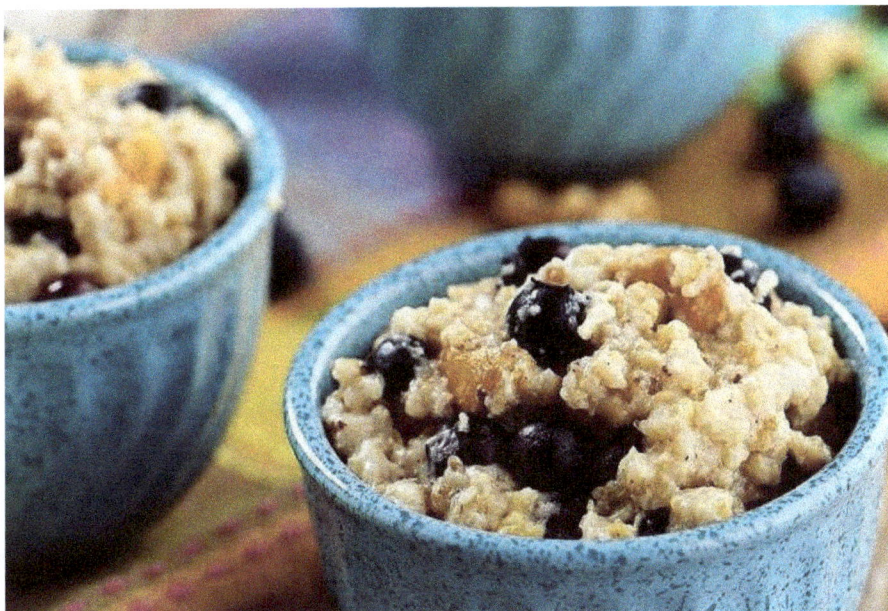

Maple Toast and Eggs

Time To Prepare: 20 Minutes
Time to Cook: 20 Minutes
Yield: Servings 6

Ingredients:

- ¼ cup butter
- ½ cup maple syrup
- 12 bacon strips, diced
- 12 big eggs
- 12 slices white bread
- Salt and pepper to taste

Directions:

1. Fry the bacon on a frying pan on moderate heat until the ‖ Fat: has rendered. Take the bacon out and place it using paper towels to drain surplus Fat.
2. Warm the maple syrup and butter until melted in a deep cooking pan. Set aside.
3. Trim the edges of the bread and flatten the slices with a rolling pin. Brush one side with the syrup mixture and press the slices into greased muffin cups.
4. Split the bacon into the muffin cups.
5. Break one egg into each cup.

6. Drizzle with salt and pepper to taste

7. Cover using foil, then bake in your oven at 4000F for about twenty minutes or until the eggs have set.

Nutritional Info: Calories: 671 ‖ Fat: 46g ‖ Carbohydrates: 44g ‖ Protein: 21g

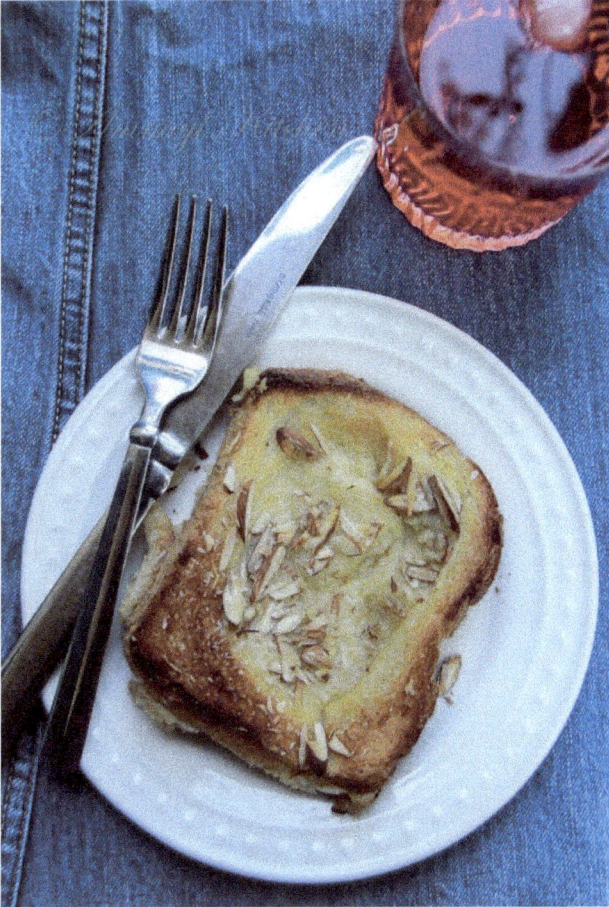

Mediterranean Frittata

Time To Prepare: five minutes

Time to Cook: twenty minutes

Yield: Servings 6

Ingredients:

- ¼ cup Black olives, chopped
- ¼ cup Feta cheese, crumbled
- ¼ cup Green olives, chopped
- ¼ cup Milk, almond or coconut
- ¼ cup Tomatoes, diced
- ¼ tsp. Black pepper
- 1 tsp. Oregano
- 1 tsp. Sea salt
- 6 Eggs
- Oil, spray or olive

Directions:

1. Heat oven to 400. Oil one eight by eight-inch baking dish.
2. Beat the milk into the eggs, and then put in other ingredients.

3. Pour all of this mixture into the baking dish and bake for 20 minutes.

Nutritional Info: Calories 107 ‖ 2 grams sugar ‖ 7g Fat ‖ 3g carbs ‖ 7 grams protein

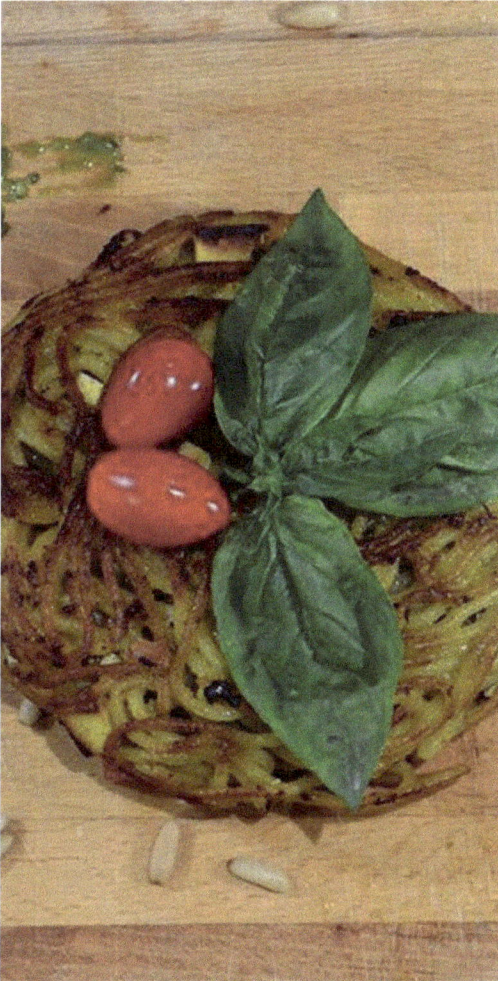

Mini Breakfast Pizza

Time To Prepare: 5 Minutes

Time to Cook: 10 Minutes

Yield: Servings 4

Ingredients:

- 4 eggs, beaten
- 2 English muffins, split and toasted
- ½ cup shredded Italian cheese
- Dried oregano leaves
- Cooking spray
- Salt and pepper to taste
- 1/3 cup commercial pizza sauce

Directions:

1. Preheat your oven to 4000F.
2. Coat a frying pan with cooking spray then heat on medium flame.
3. Flavour the eggs with salt and pepper to taste and pour into the frying pan. As the eggs start to set, pull the eggs across the pan with an inverted turner. Carry on cooking and folding the egg. Set aside.
4. Spread pizza sauce uniformly on English muffin halves and top with eggs and cheese.

5. Put on a baking sheet then bake for five minutes.

6. Decorate using oregano last.

Nutritional Info: Calories: 282 ‖ Fat: 13g ‖ Carbohydrates: 25g ‖ Protein: 17g

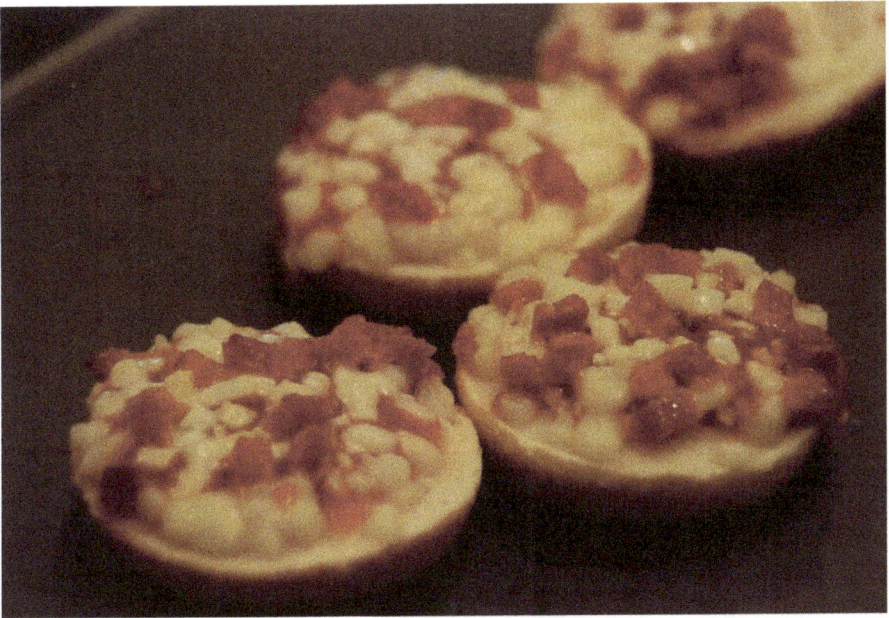

Mushroom Crêpes

Time To Prepare: 1 hour thirty minutes

Time to Cook: thirty minutes

Yield: Servings 6

Ingredients:

- 2 eggs
- ½ cup all-purpose flour
- For the filling
- 3 tablespoons all-purpose flour
- 2 cups of cremini mushrooms, cut
- ½ cup Parmesan cheese, grated
- ¾ cup milk
- 3 garlic cloves, minced
- 2 tablespoons of parsley (chopped)
- 6 slices of deli-cut cooked lean ham
- Freshly ground pepper
- 1/4 teaspoon salt
- 1/4 teaspoon of salt
- 3/4 cup milk
- 3/4 cup chicken broth
- 1/8 teaspoon cayenne
- 1/8 teaspoon nutmeg

Directions:

1. Put and mix the salt and flour in a container. In another container, whisk the eggs and milk. Slowly mix the two mixtures until the desired smoothness is achieved. Leave for fifteen minutes.

2. Spray a frying pan using non-stick cooking spray and put on moderate heat. Mix the batter a little. Put in 1/4 of the batter into the frying pan. Tilt the frying pan to make a thin and even crêpe. Cook for a couple of minutes or until the bottom is golden and the top is set. Flip and cook for twenty seconds. Move to a plate.

3. Repeat the steps with the rest of the batter. Loosely cover the cooked crêpes using plastic wrap.

4. For the filling. Combine all ingredients for filling in a deep cooking pan on moderate heat – flour, milk, cayenne, nutmeg, and pepper. Constantly whisk until thick or around seven minutes. Take off the stove. Mix in a tablespoon of parsley and cheese. Loosely cover to keep warm.

5. Spray a frying pan using non-stick cooking spray and put on moderate heat. Cook the garlic and mushrooms. Sprinkle with salt. Cook for about six minutes or until the mushrooms are tender. Put in 2 tablespoons of sherry. Cook for about 2 minutes. Take off the stove. Put in the remaining parsley and stir.

6. Place the crêpes side by side on a flat surface. Spread a tablespoon of the sauce and 2 tablespoons of the cooked mushrooms. Roll up the crêpes and move them to a greased baking dish. Put all the sauce on top. Bake using your oven at 450°F for fifteen minutes.

Nutritional Info: Calories: 232 kcal ‖ Protein: 16.51 g ‖ Fat: 10.8 g ‖ Carbohydrates: 16.25 g

Nutty Oats Pudding

Time To Prepare: five minutes

Time to Cook: 0 minutes

Yield: Servings 3 -5

Ingredients:

- ¼ cup dry milk
- ¼ cup rolled oats
- ½ cup of water
- 1 ½ tablespoon natural peanut butter
- 1 tablespoon yogurt, fat-free
- 1 teaspoon peanuts, finely chopped

Directions:

1. Using a microwaveable-safe container, put together peanut butter and dry milk. Whisk well. Put in in water to achieve a smooth consistency. Put in in oats.
2. Cover container using plastic wrap. Create a small hole for the steam to escape.
3. Put inside the microwave oven for a minute on high powder.
4. Continue heating, this time on medium power for 90 seconds. Allow to sit for five minutes.

5. To serve, spoon an equal amount of cereals in a container top with peanuts and yogurt.

Nutritional Info: Calories: 70 kcal ‖ Protein: 4.25 g ‖ Fat: 3.83 g ‖ Carbohydrates: 6.78 g

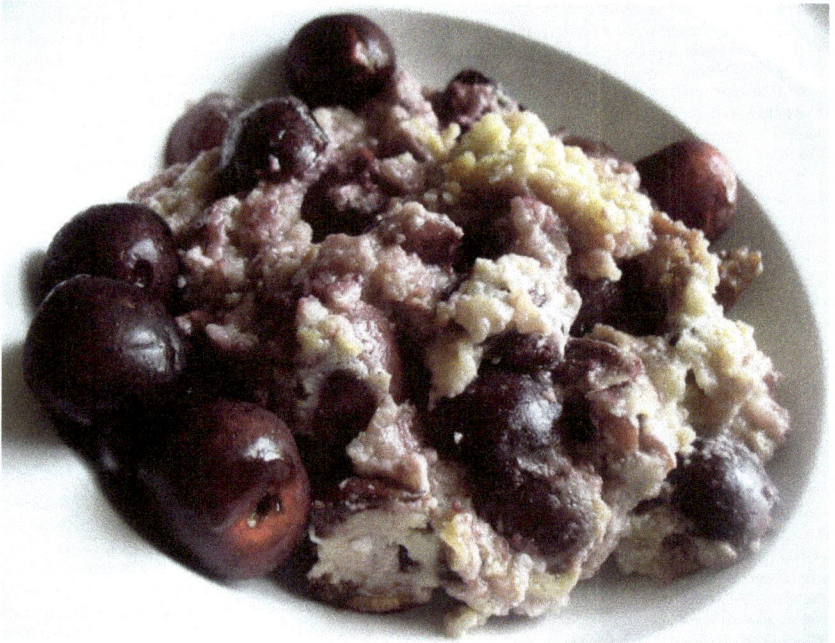

Oat Porridge with Cherry & Coconut

Time To Prepare: ten minutes

Time to Cook: 0 minutes

Yield: Servings 3

Ingredients:

- 1 ½ cups regular oats
- 3 cups coconut milk
- 3 tbsp. raw cacao
- 4 tbsp. chia seed
- A pinch of stevia, optional
- Coconut shavings
- Dark chocolate shavings
- Fresh or frozen tart cherries
- Maple syrup, to taste (not necessary)

Directions:

1. Mix the oats, milk, stevia, and cacao in a moderate-sized deep cooking pan on moderate heat and bring to its boiling point. Reduce the heat, then simmer until the oats are cooked to desired doneness.

2. Split the porridge among 3 serving bowls and top with dark chocolate and coconut shavings, cherries, and a little sprinkle of maple syrup.

Nutritional Info: Calories: 343 kcal ‖ Protein: 15.64 g ‖ Fat: 12.78 g ‖ Carbohydrates: 41.63 g

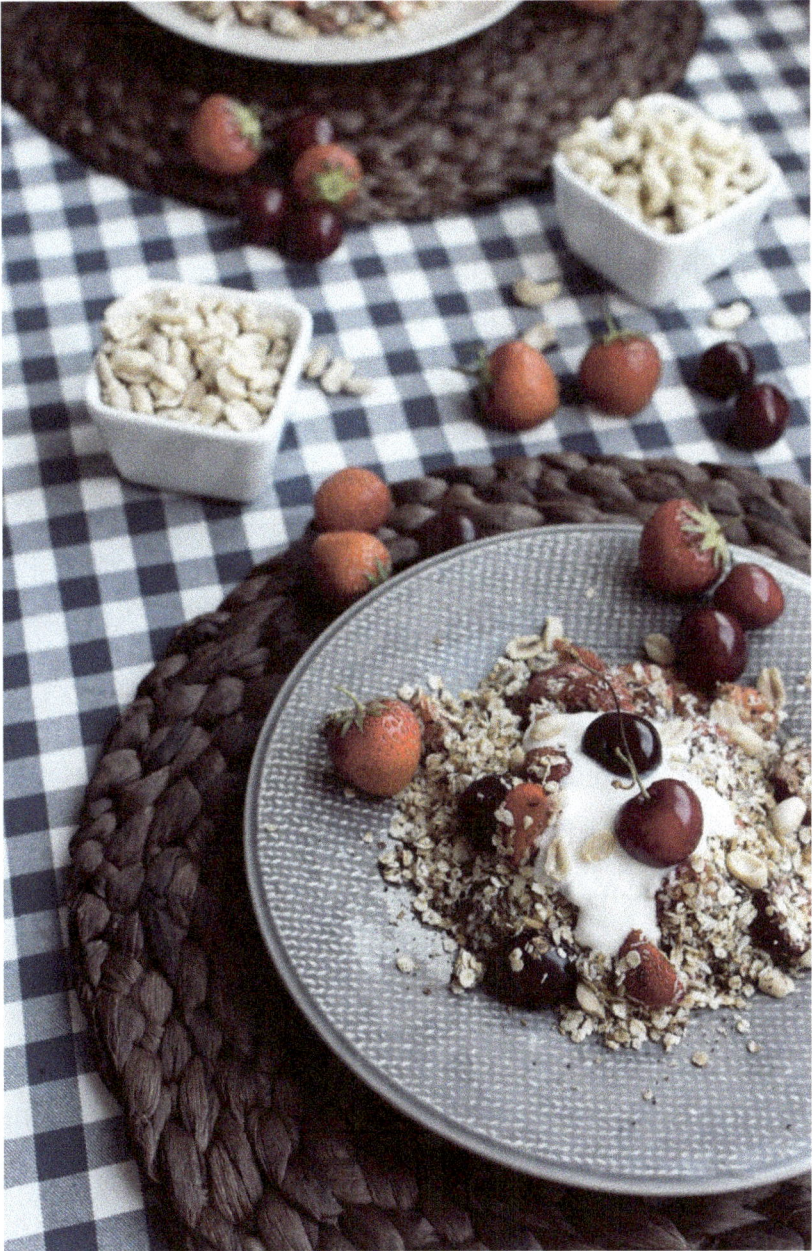

SMOOTHIES AND DRINKS

Lemon Ginger Iced Tea

Time To Prepare: five minutes

Time to Cook: ten minutes

Yield: Servings 2-3

Ingredients:

- ¼ teaspoon turmeric
- 1 tablespoon fresh lemon juice or to taste (not necessary)
- 1 tablespoon maple syrup
- 2 – 3 lemon slices
- 2 inches fresh ginger, peeled, thinly cut or to taste
- 3-4 cups water
- A pinch ground cinnamon

Directions:

1. Pour water into a deep cooking pan. Put in ginger, turmeric, lemon slices, and cinnamon. Put the deep cooking pan on moderate heat.
2. Cover and simmer for eight - ten minutes.

3. Strain and pour into a jar. Place the maple syrup, and lemon juice, then stir. Chill for eight – 10 hours.

4. Stir thoroughly. Pour into glasses before you serve.

Nutritional Info: Calories: 55 kcal ‖ Protein: 2.32 g ‖ Fat: 2.13 g ‖ Carbohydrates: 7.47 g

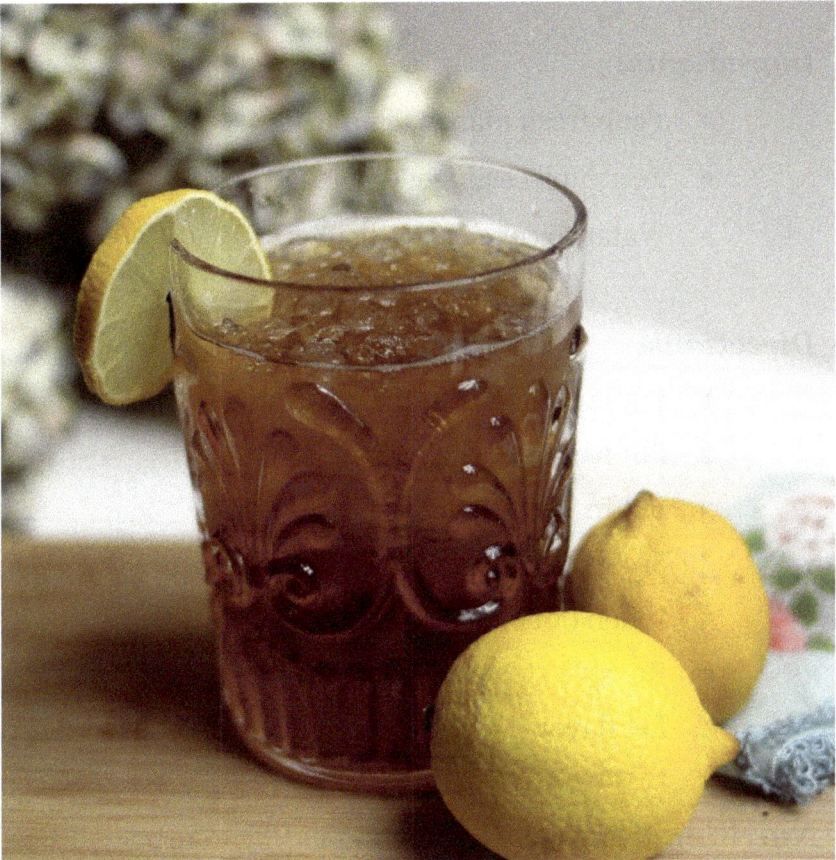

Mango and Ginger Infused Water

Time To Prepare: five minutes
Time to Cook: five minutes
Yield: Servings 4

Ingredients:

- 1 cup fresh mango, chopped
- 2-inch piece ginger, peeled, cubed
- Water to cover ingredients

Directions:

1. Put ingredients in the mesh steamer basket.
2. Put basket in the instant pot.
3. Put in water to immerse contents.
4. Secure the lid. Cook on HIGH pressure five minutes.
5. When done, depressurize swiftly.
6. Remove steamer basket. Discard cooked produce.
7. Let flavored water cool. Chill completely and serve.

Nutritional Info: Calories: 209 ‖ Fat: 1g ‖ Carbohydrates: 51g ‖ Protein: 2g

Mango Tomato Smoothie

Time To Prepare: five minutes

Time to Cook: 0 minutes

Yield: Servings 4

Ingredients:

- 1 cup almond milk
- 2 cups chopped cilantro
- 2 cups pineapple chunks
- 2 mangoes, peeled, pitted
- 4 Campari tomatoes, chopped
- 6 cups fresh baby spinach

Directions:

1. Combine all ingredients into a blender and blend until the desired smoothness is achieved.
2. Pour into 4 tall glasses before you serve.

Nutritional Info: Calories: 395 kcal ‖ Protein: 13.1 g ‖ Fat: 8.19 g ‖ Carbohydrates: 73.65 g

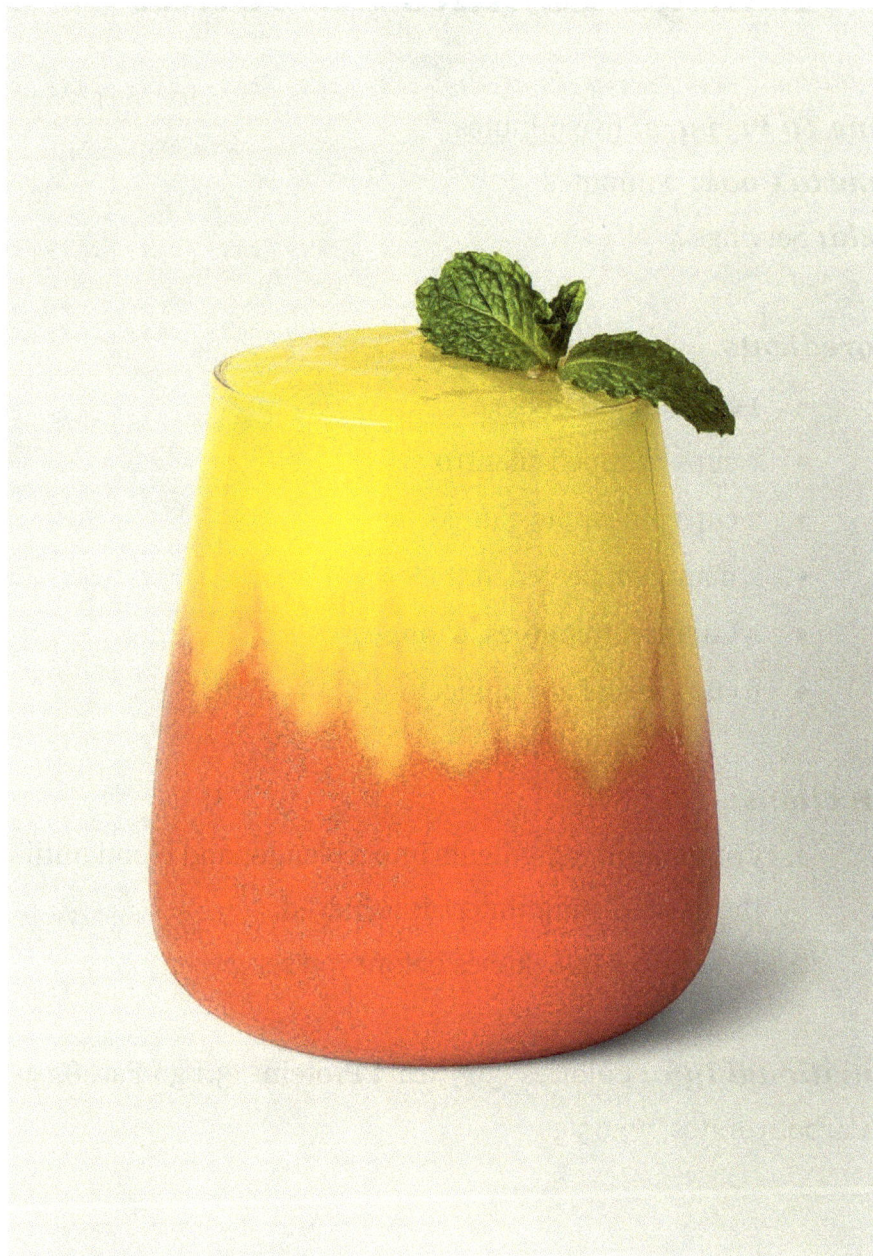

Mixed Fruit & Nut Milkshake

Time To Prepare: five minutes

Time to Cook: 0 minutes

Yield: Servings 2

Ingredients:

- 1 tbsp. of honey
- 1/2 cup of almond milk
- 1½ grapefruit; peeled and chopped
- 1/2½ inch piece of ginger, minced
- 12 strawberries
- 2 tbsp. of chopped almonds
- juice of 1 orange

Directions:

1. Put everything but the strawberries in a blender until the desired smoothness is achieved.
2. Put in in the strawberries and blend until pureed, serving in a tall glass.

Nutritional Info: Calories: 140 kcal ‖ Protein: 5.89 g ‖ Fat: 5.84 g ‖ Carbohydrates: 17.36 g

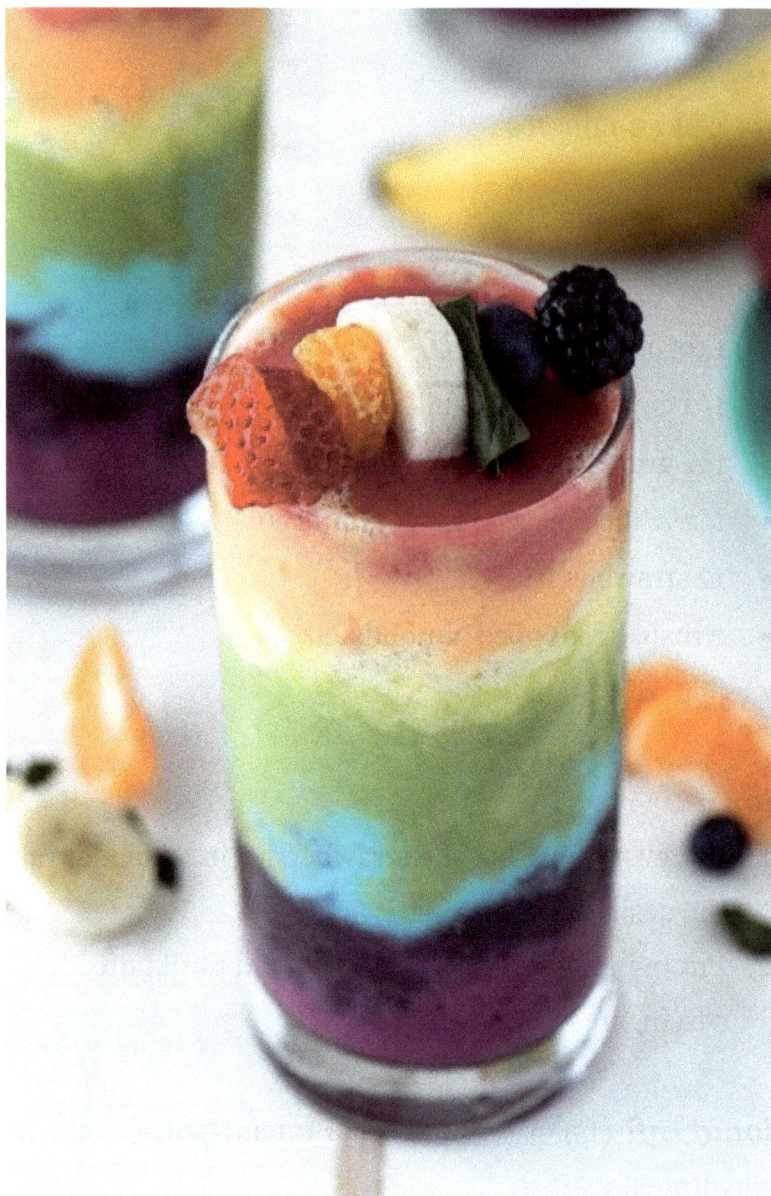

Parsley Ginger Green Juice

Time To Prepare: five minutes

Time to Cook: 0 minutes

Yield: Servings 2

Ingredients:

- 2 cucumbers, chopped
- 2 green apples, cored
- 2 lemons, peeled, halved
- 4 cups chopped parsley
- 4 cups chopped spinach
- 4 inches fresh ginger, peeled, cut
- 6 stalks celery, chopped

Directions:

1. Juice together all the ingredients in a juicer.
2. Pour into 2 glasses before you serve.

Nutritional Info: Calories: 239 kcal ‖ Protein: 10.74 g ‖ Fat: 5.08 g ‖ Carbohydrates: 44.86 g

Peach And Raspberry Lemonade

Time To Prepare: five minutes
Time to Cook: five minutes
Yield: Servings 4

Ingredients:

- ½ cup fresh raspberries
- 1 cup fresh peaches, chopped
- Water to cover ingredients
- Zest and juice of 1 lemon

Directions:

1. Put ingredients in mesh basket for instant pot. Put in pot.
2. Put in water to barely cover the fruit.
3. Secure the lid. Cook on HIGH pressure five minutes.
4. When done, depressurize swiftly.
5. Remove steamer basket. Discard cooked produce.
6. Let flavored water cool. Chill completely before you serve.

Nutritional Info: Calories: 77 ‖ Fat: 0g ‖ Carbohydrates: 19g ‖ Protein: 0g

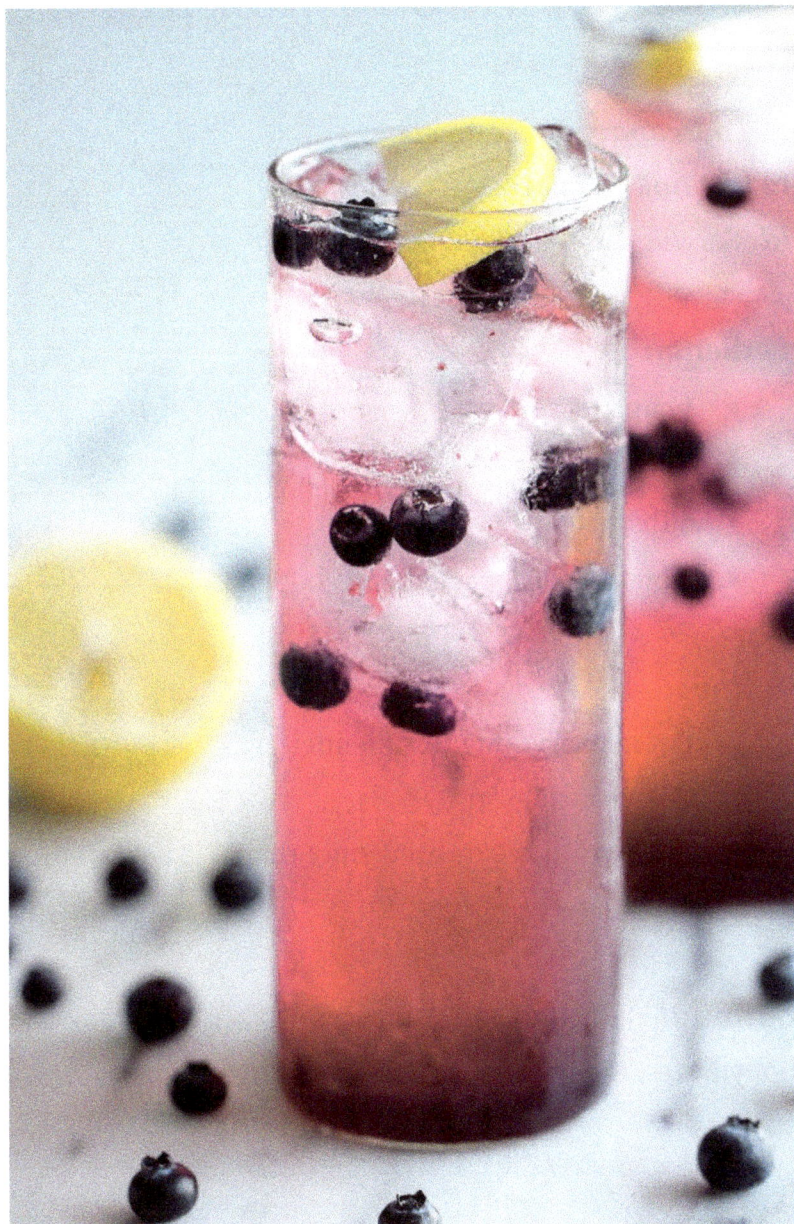

Peach Maple Smoothie

Time To Prepare: ten minutes

Time to Cook: 0 minutes

Yield: Servings 1

Ingredients:

- 1 cup fat-free yogurt
- 1 cup ice
- 2 tbsp. maple syrup
- 4 big peaches, peeled and chopped

Directions:

1. Put in everything to a blender jug.
2. Cover the jug firmly.
3. Blend until the desired smoothness is achieved. Serve and enjoy!

Nutritional Info: Calories: 125 ‖ Fat: 0.4 g ‖ Protein: 5.6 g ‖ Carbohydrates: 8 g ‖ Fiber: 2.3 g

SIDES

Onion and Orange Healthy Salad

Time To Prepare: ten minutes

Time to Cook: 0 minutes

Yield: Servings 3

Ingredients:

- ¼ cup of fresh chives, chopped
- 1 cup olive oil
- 1 red onion, thinly cut
- 1 teaspoon of dried oregano
- 3 tablespoon of red wine vinegar
- 6 big orange
- 6 tablespoon of olive oil
- Ground black pepper

Directions:

1. Peel the orange and cut each of them in 4-5 crosswise slices
2. Move the oranges to a shallow dish

3. Sprinkle vinegar, olive oil and drizzle oregano

4. Toss

5. Chill for thirty minutes

6. Position cut onion and black olives on top

7. Garnish with an additional drizzle of chives and a fresh grind of pepper

8. Serve and enjoy!

Nutritional Info: ‖ Calories: 120 ‖ Fat: 6g ‖ Carbohydrates: 20g ‖ Protein: 2g

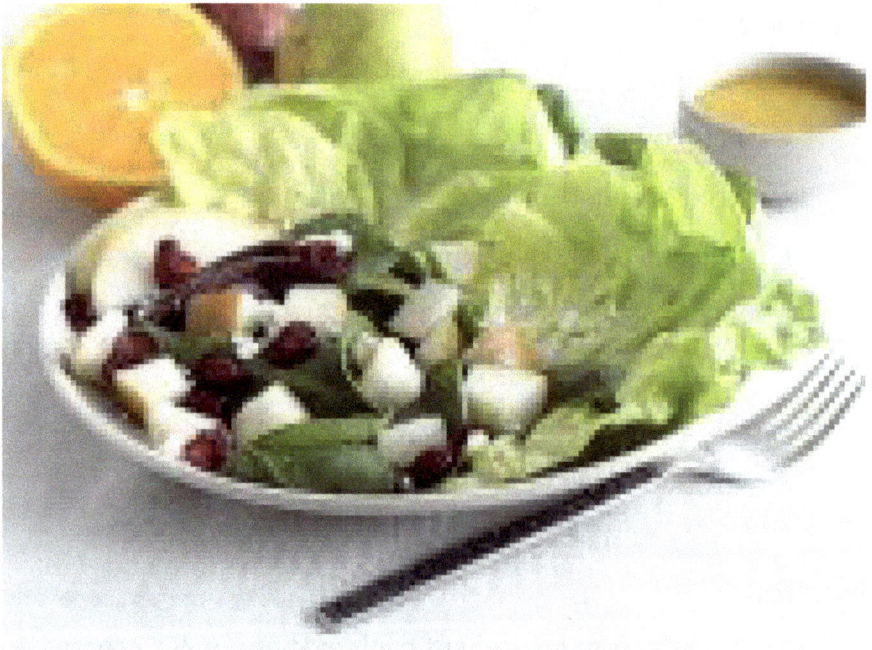

Parmesan Roasted Broccoli

Time To Prepare: ten minutes

Time to Cook: twenty minutes

Yield: Servings 6

Ingredients:

- ½ teaspoon of Italian seasoning
- 1 tablespoon of lemon juice
- 1 tablespoon parsley, chopped
- 3 tablespoons of olive oil
- 3 tablespoons of vegan parmesan, grated
- 4 cups of broccoli florets
- Pepper and salt to taste

Directions:

1. Preheat the oven to 450 degrees F. Apply cooking spray on your pan.
2. Keep the broccoli florets in a freezer bag.
3. Now put in the Italian seasoning, olive oil, pepper, and salt.
4. Seal your bag. Shake it. Coat well.
5. Pour your broccoli on the pan. It must be in a single layer.
6. Bake for about twenty minutes. Stir midway through.

7. Take out from the oven. Drizzle parsley and parmesan.

8. Sprinkle some lemon juice.

9. You can decorate with lemon wedges if you wish.

Nutritional Info: Calories 96 ‖ Carbohydrates: 4g ‖ Cholesterol: 2mg ‖ Total Fat: 8g ‖ Protein: 2g ‖ Sugar: 1g ‖ Fiber: 1g ‖ Sodium: 58mg ‖ Potassium: 191mg

Quinoa Salad

Time To Prepare: ten minutes

Time to Cook: 0 minutes

Yield: Servings 2

Ingredients:

- ¼ tsp sea salt
- ½ cup quinoa (uncooked)
- 1 carrot
- 1 tbsp. apple cider vinegar
- 1 tbsp. flaxseed oil
- 2 brussels sprouts

Directions:

1. Wash quinoa meticulously.
2. Dice the carrots and brussels sprouts to minuscule pieces.
3. Cook the quinoa based on the instruction on the packaging.
4. Mix flaxseed oil, sea salt, and apple cider vinegar.
5. Sauté brussels sprouts and carrots on a small amount of olive oil for a few minutes.
6. After both brussels sprouts and carrots, and quinoa are ready, combine them all in a container.

7. Put in the dressing and mix meticulously.

8. Serve warm.

Nutritional Info: ‖ Calories: 280 kcal ‖ Protein: 10.15 g ‖ Fat: 12.52 g ‖ Carbohydrates: 31.99 g

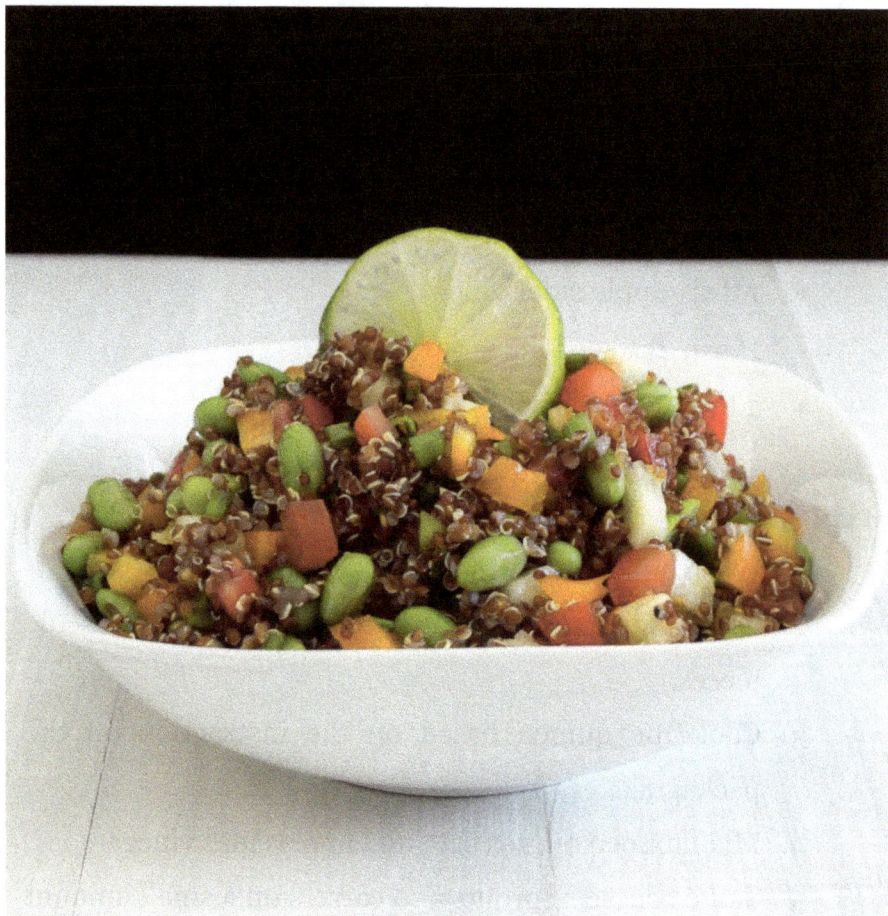

Red Cabbage with Cheese

Time To Prepare: five minutes

Time to Cook: twelve minutes

Yield: Servings 4

Ingredients:

- ¼ cup & 1 tbsp. of extra virgin olive oil
- ¼ tsp of freshly ground pepper
- ¼ tsp of salt
- 1 cup of walnuts
- 1 Tbsp. of crumbled blue cheese
- 1 tbsp. of Dijon mustard
- 1 tsp of butter
- 2 thinly cut scallions
- 3 tbsp. of pure maple syrup
- 3 tbsp. of red wine vinegar
- 8 cups of red cabbage, thinly cut

Directions:

For the vinaigrette:

1. Combine the blue cheese, ¼ cup of olive oil, mustard, vinegar, salt, and pepper in a food processor or blender until the mixture has a creamy consistency.

For the salad:

1. Put a parchment paper near the stove.
2. Heat 1 tbsp. Of oil on moderate heat in a moderate-sized frying pan and mix in the walnuts, cooking them for approximately 2 minutes.
3. Now mix salt and pepper, sprinkle maple syrup and cook for approximately three to five minutes while stirring the mixture up to the nuts are uniformly coated.
4. Move to the paper and pour the rest of the syrup over them using a spoon. Separate the nuts and cool down for approximately five minutes.
5. In a big container, put in the cabbage and scallions and toss them with the vinaigrette. Put in the walnuts and blue cheese as toppings.

Nutritional Info: Calories 232 ‖ Fat: 19 gram Saturated ‖ Fat: 4 gram ‖ Sodium: 267 gram ‖ Carbs: 12 gram ‖ Fiber: 2 gram sugar ‖ 8 gram Added sugar 5 gram ‖ Protein: 4 gram

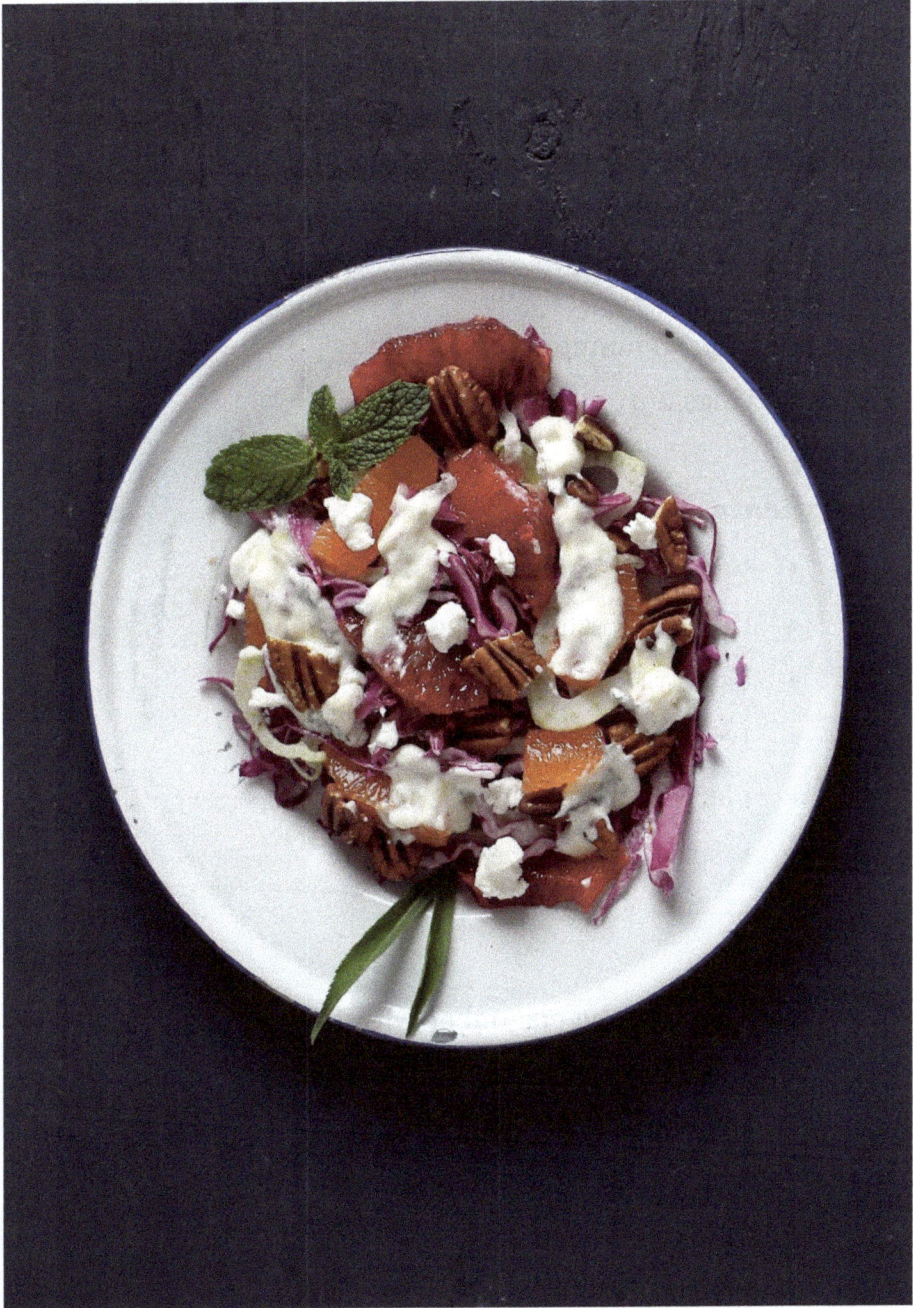

SAUCES AND DRESSINGS

Herby Raita

Time To Prepare: ten minutes

Time to Cook: 0 minutes

Yield: Servings 2-4

Ingredients:

- ¼ cup of freshly chopped mint
- ¼ tsp of freshly ground black pepper
- ½ tsp of sea salt
- 1 cup of Greek yogurt
- 1 large-sized cucumber, shredded
- 1 tsp of lemon juice

Directions:

1. Combine the cucumber with ¼ tsp of salt in a sieve and leave to drain for fifteen minutes. Shake to release any surplus liquid and move to a kitchen towel. Squeeze out as much liquid as you can using the paper towel.

2. Put the cucumber into a medium container then mix in the rest of the ingredients until well blended.

3. Put in your fridge for minimum 2 hours to keep its freshness. Best consume with spicy foods as it could relief the spiciness.

Nutritional Info: ‖ Calories: 69 kcal ‖ Protein: 4.33 g ‖ Fat: 3.66 g ‖ Carbohydrates: 4.93 g

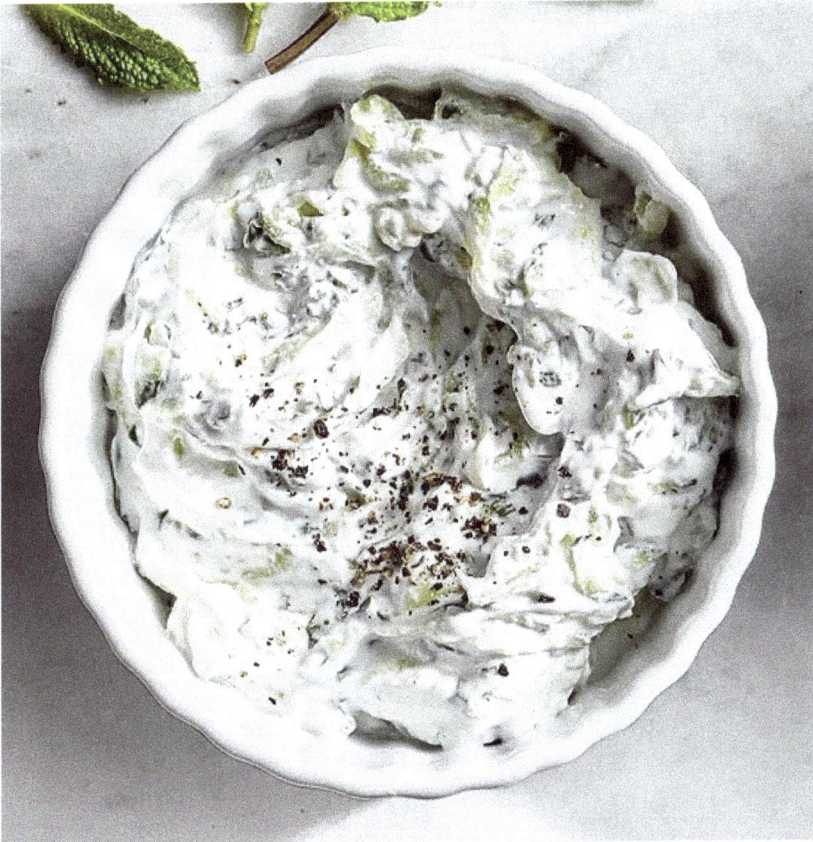

Homemade Ginger Dressing

Time To Prepare: ten minutes

Time to Cook: 0 minutes

Yield: Servings 2-4

Ingredients:

- ¼ cup of chopped celery
- ¼ cup of honey or maple syrup
- ¼ cup of water
- ½ cup of chopped carrots
- ½ tsp of white pepper
- 1 cup of chopped onion
- 1 cup of extra-virgin olive oil
- 1 tsp of freshly minced garlic
- 1 tsp of kosher salt
- 2 ½ tbsp. of unsalted, gluten-free soy sauce
- 2 tbsp. of ketchup
- 2/3 cup of rice vinegar
- 6 tbsp. of freshly grated ginger

Directions:

1. Put the onion, ginger, celery, carrots, and garlic into a blender. Blend until the mixture are fine but still lumpy from the small vegetable chunks.
2. Put in in the vinegar, water, ketchup, soy sauce, honey or maple syrup, lemon juice, salt, and pepper. Pulse until the ingredients are well blended.
3. Slowly put in the oil while blending, until everything is thoroughly combined. The mixture must be runny but still grainy.
4. Serve with a winter salad.

Nutritional Info: ‖ Calories: 389 kcal ‖ Protein: 2.71 g ‖ Fat: 32.08 g ‖ Carbohydrates: 22.14 g

SNACKS

Energetic Oat Bars

Time To Prepare: ten minutes

Time to Cook: twenty-five minutes

Yield: Servings 6

Ingredients:

- ½ cup of gluten-free rolled oats
- ¾ cup fresh blueberries
- 1 peeled and mashed banana
- 1 tbsp. of chopped walnuts
- 1 tbsp. of fresh pomegranate juice
- 1 tbsp. of sunflower seeds
- 2 tbsp. of flax seeds
- 2 tbsp. of pitted and chopped finely dates
- 2 tbsp. of raisins

Directions:

1. Set the oven to 350F. Lightly, oil an 8-inch baking dish.

2. In a huge mixing container, put all ingredients and mix till well blended.

3. Put the mixture into the readied baking dish uniformly.

4. Bake for approximately twenty-five minutes. Remove from the oven then cool.

5. Using a knife, split the bars into the size your desired pieces then serve.

Nutritional Info: ‖ Calories: 88 ‖ Fat: 2.3g ‖ Carbohydrates: 18.2g ‖ Protein: 2.3g ‖ Fiber: 2.8g

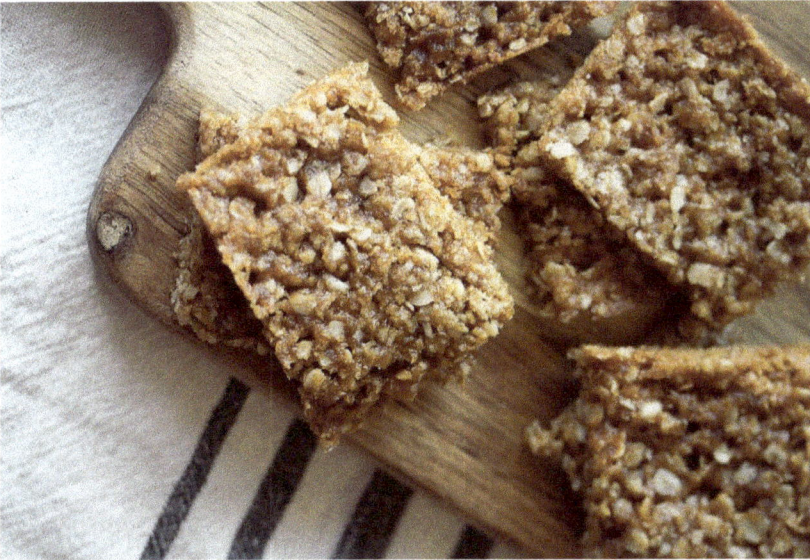

Energy Dates Balls

Time To Prepare: ten minutes

Time to Cook: twenty-five minutes

Yield: Servings 7

Ingredients:

- ¼ cup of fresh lemon juice
- ½ cup of shredded sweetened coconut
- 1 cup of pitted and chopped dates
- 1 cup of toasted almonds

Directions:

1. Coat a big baking sheet using a parchment paper. Keep aside.
2. Use a food processor to add almonds and pulse till chopped crudely.
3. Put in dates and lemon juice and pulse till a tender dough forms.
4. Make equal sized balls from the mixture.
5. In a shallow, dish place shredded coconut.
6. Roll the balls in shredded coconut uniformly.
7. Place the balls onto the baking sheet in a single layer.
8. Place in your fridge to set completely before you serve.

Nutritional Info: ‖ Calories: 173 ‖ Fat: 7.9g ‖ Carbohydrates: 23g ‖ Protein: 3.8g ‖ Fiber: 4.3g

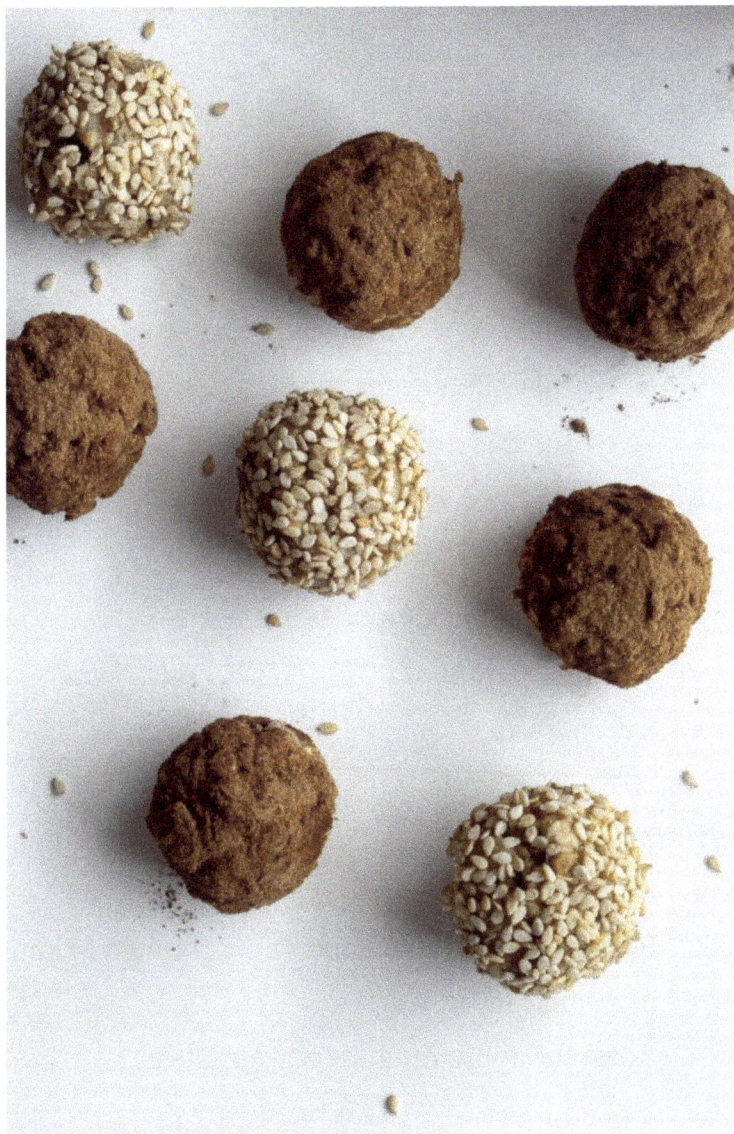

Flavorsome Almonds

Time To Prepare: ten minutes

Time to Cook: fifteen minutes

Yield: Servings 8

Ingredients:

- ¼ tsp. of cayenne pepper
- ¼ tsp. of ground cumin
- ½ tsp. of chili powder
- ½ tsp. of ground cinnamon
- 1 tbsp. of filtered water
- 1 tsp. of extra-virgin olive oil
- 2 cups of whole almonds
- 3 tbsp. of raw honey
- Salt, to taste

Directions:

1. Preheat your oven to 350 degrees F.
2. Position the almonds onto a big rimmed baking sheet in a single layer.
3. Roast for approximately ten minutes.

4. In the meantime, in a microwave-safe container, put in honey and microwave on Hugh for approximately half a minute.

5. Remove from microwave and mix in oil and water.

6. In a small container, combine all spices.

7. Take away the almonds from the oven, put in it into the container of honey mixture, and stir until blended well.

8. Move the almond mixture onto the baking sheet in a single layer.

9. Drizzle with spice mixture uniformly.

10. Roast for approximately 3-4 minutes.

11. Take off from oven and keep aside to cool to room temperature and serve.

12. You can preserve these roasted almonds in an airtight jar.

Nutritional Info: ‖ Calories: 168 ‖ Fat: 12.5g ‖ Carbohydrates: 11.8g ‖ Protein: 5.1g ‖ Fiber: 3.1g

Flourless & Flaky Muffin Munchies

Time To Prepare: twenty-five minutes
Time to Cook: twenty minutes
Yield: Servings 4

Ingredients:

- ⅛-tsp baking soda
- ¼-cup peanut butter or allergy-friendly substitution
- ¼-cup pure maple syrup or honey
- ¼-tsp salt
- ½-cup quick oats or quinoa flakes, loosely packed
- ¾-tsp baking powder
- 1-cup white beans, cooked
- 1-pc medium mashed banana, very ripe
- 2-tsp pure vanilla extract
- A handful of mini chocolate chips, crushed walnuts, shredded coconut, pinch cinnamon, etc. (not necessary)

Directions:

1. Preheat your oven to 350 F. Coat 8-muffin cups with glassine.

2. Mix all the ingredients in your blender. Blend to a smooth consistency. Pour the mixture into the muffin cups at ⅔ full.

3. Place the cups in your oven, and bake for about twenty minutes.

4. Allow the muffins to sit and cool for about twenty minutes.

Nutritional Info: ‖ Calories: 119 ‖ Fat: 3.9g ‖ Protein: 8.9g ‖ Sodium: 102mg ‖ Total Carbohydrates: 14.4g ‖ Fiber: 2.5g ‖ Net Carbohydrates: 11.9g

Ginger Flour Banana Ginger Bars

Time To Prepare: ten minutes
Time to Cook: forty minutes
Yield: Servings 4-6

Ingredients:

- 1 ½ tbsp. Grated ginger
- 1 cup Coconut flour
- 1 tsp. Baking soda
- 1 tsp. Ground cardamom
- 1/3 cup Honey or maple syrup
- 1/3 cup melted butter
- 2 big Ripe bananas
- 2 tsp. Apple cider vinegar
- 2 tsp. Cinnamon
- 6 medium While eggs

Directions:

1. Preheat your oven to 350°F.
2. Coat a glass baking dish using parchment paper. If you do not have any paper, just grease the pan.

3. Put all the ingredients apart from the baking soda and apple cider vinegar through a food processor and pulse until it's all mixed up.
4. Now put in the last two ingredients and blitz once before pouring the mix into the glass dish.
5. Bake up to a toothpick inserted into the center comes out clean. This usually takes forty minutes.

Nutritional Info: ‖ Calories: 1407 kcal ‖ Protein: 42.18 g ‖ Fat: 100.26 g ‖ Carbohydrates: 88.33 g

Ginger Turmeric ‖ Protein: Bars

Time To Prepare: ten minutes + 20 cooling time

Time to Cook: twenty-five minutes

Yield: Servings 7

Ingredients:

- ½ cup coconut
- 1 cup cashews
- 1 scoop turmeric Protein bone broth
- 1 Tbsp. ginger
- 1/3 cup sunflower butter
- 2 Tbsp. maple syrup

Directions:

1. Put in coconut pieces and cashews to a blender or food processor. Use the pulse option to obtain a coarse mixture.

2. Put in butter, broth, maple syrup, and ginger and pulse the mixture to make a coarse, yet even and fairly sticky mass.

3. Evenly put the mixture to a baking pan (8x8 inches) with your hands or a spoon. Push tightly to the baking pan.

4. Bring it in a fridge and allow it to cool for about twenty minutes.

5. Chop the mixture into even squares.

6. You can consume instantly or store in a glass container in the refrigerator (up to 7 days).

Nutritional Info: 107 kcal ‖ Protein: 1.15 g ‖ Fat: 9.59 g ‖ Carbohydrates: 4.63 g

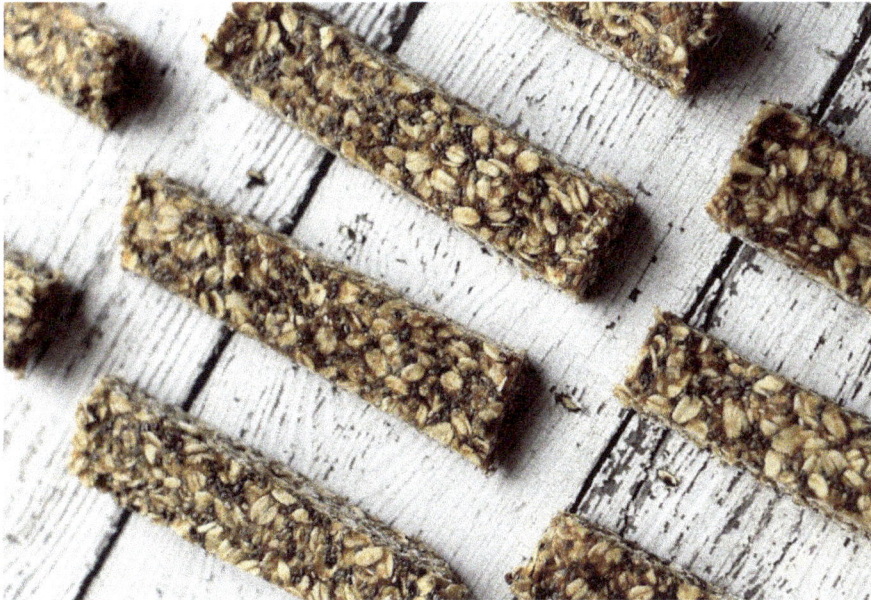

Hummus Deviled Eggs

Time To Prepare: ten minutes
Time to Cook: 0 minutes
Yield: Servings 6

Ingredients:

- ½ cup hummus
- 6 hard-boiled eggs
- Paprika

Directions:

1. Cut the hardboiled eggs in half along the length and remove the yolk.
2. Fill the egg whites with hummus and drizzle with paprika before you serve.

Nutritional Info: ‖ Calories: 179 kcal ‖ Protein: 11.03 g ‖ Fat: 12.41 g ‖ Carbohydrates: 5.14 g

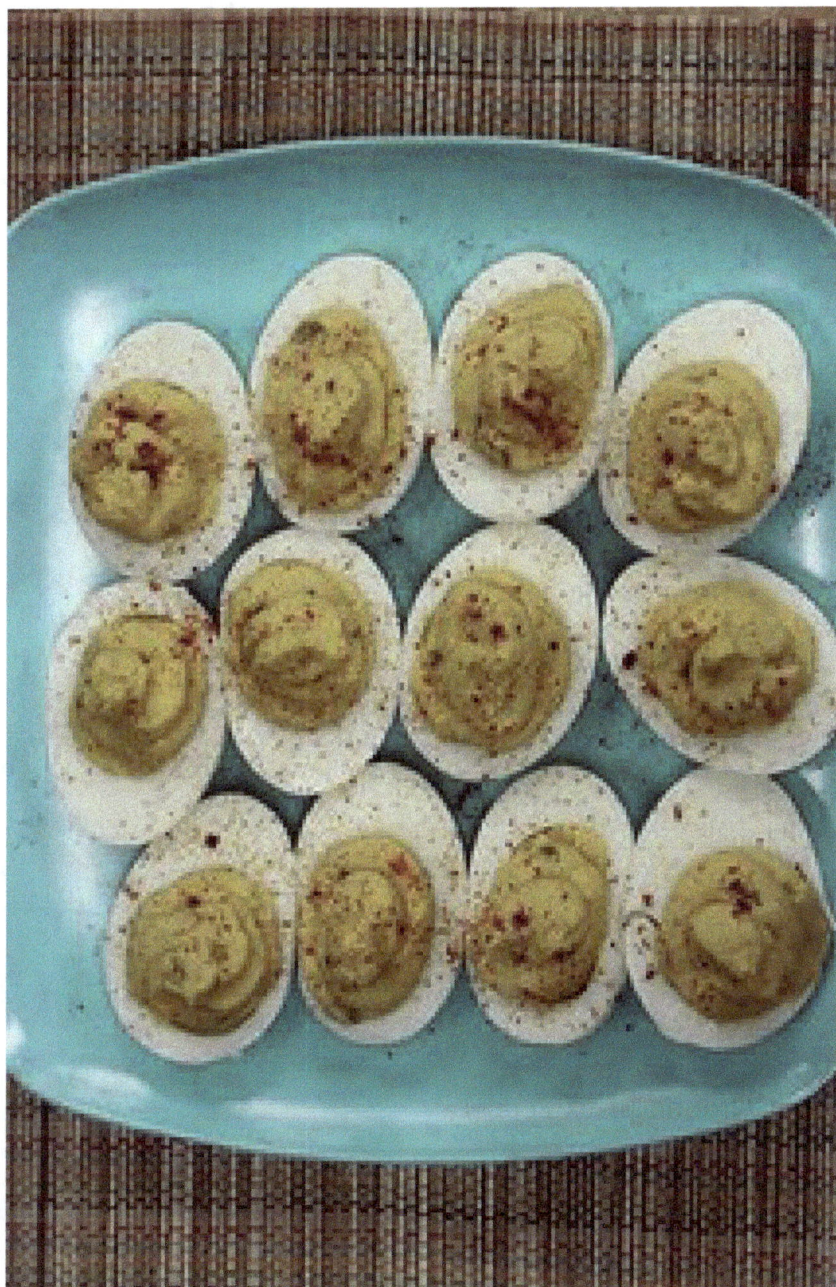

SOUPS AND STEWS

Hungarian Lentil Soup

Time To Prepare: fifteen minutes

Time to Cook: 2 hours

Yield: Servings 8

Ingredients:

- 7 Cups Chicken Stock
- 3 Carrots (Diced)
- 2 Stalks Celery (Diced)
- 1 Teaspoon Garlic (Minced)
- 2 Bay Leaves
- 1 Sprig Fresh Parsley (Chopped)
- 2 Tablespoons Olive Oil
- 2 Large Onions (Cubed)
- Salt
- Ground Black Pepper
- 1½ Cups Lentils (Soaked, Rinsed, Drained)
- ½ Teaspoon Paprika
- ½ Cup Grated Parmesan Cheese
- 3½ Cups Crushed Tomatoes

- 3/4 Cup White Wine

Directions:

1. Sauté onions in oil until shiny and put in garlic, paprika, celery, and carrots, cooking for about ten minutes.
2. Mix in tomatoes, chicken stock, lentils, bay leaves, seasoning, and wine to boil.
3. Cook until the lentils are soft.
4. Top with parsley and Parmesan before you serve.

Nutritional Info: Calories: 258 kcal ‖ Carbohydrates: 34 g ‖ Fat: 6 g ‖ Protein: 14 g

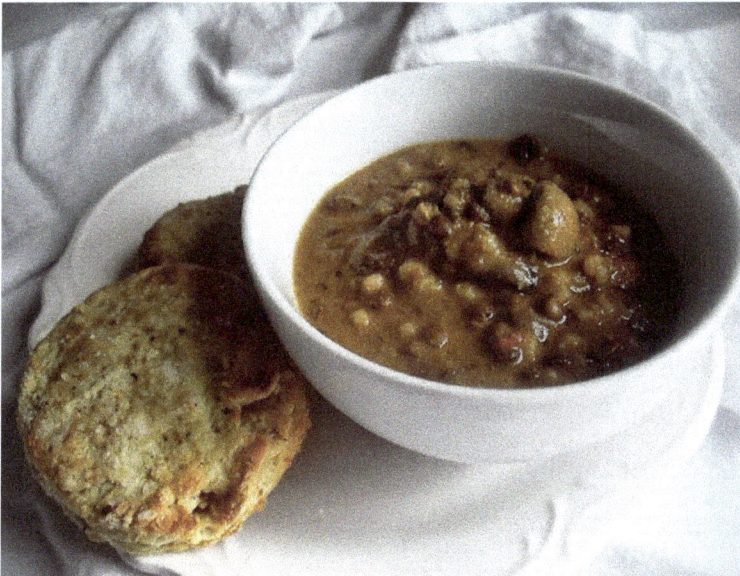

Italian Beef Soup

Time To Prepare: ten minutes

Time to Cook: 4 hours

Yield: Servings 6

Ingredients:

- ½ cup diced tomatoes
- ½ cup shredded mozzarella cheese
- 1 cup beef broth
- 1 cup heavy cream
- 1 pound lean ground beef
- 1 tablespoon Italian seasoning
- 1 yellow onion, chopped
- 2 cloves garlic, chopped
- Salt & pepper, to taste

Directions:

1. Put in all the ingredients to a slow cooker minus the heavy cream and mozzarella cheese. Cook on high for 4 hours.
2. Warm the heavy cream, and then put in the warmed cream and cheese to the soup. Stir thoroughly before you serve.

Nutritional Info: Calories: 241 ‖ Carbohydrates: 4g ‖ Fiber: 1g Net ‖ Carbohydrates: 3g ‖ Fat: 14g ‖ Protein: 25g

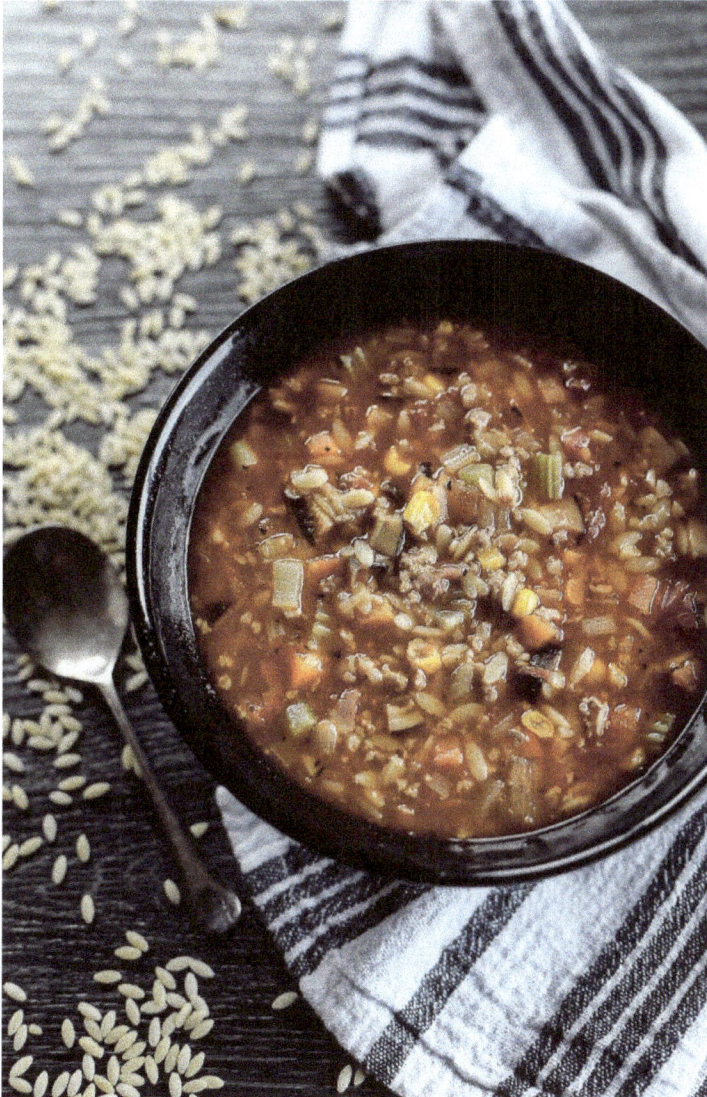

Italian Modena Soup

Time To Prepare: two minutes
Time to Cook: 8 minutes
Yield: Servings 4

Ingredients:

- ½ cup Parmigiano-Reggiano cheese, shaved
- ½ teaspoon crushed chili
- 1 cup water
- 1 onion, chopped
- 1 tablespoon Italian seasonings
- 16 ounces Cotechino di Modena, cut
- 2 cups tomatoes, purée
- 2 tablespoons olive oil
- 3 cups roasted vegetable broth
- Sea salt and ground black pepper, to taste

Directions:

1. Push the "Sauté" button to heat up your Instant Pot. Once hot, heat the oil and sauté the onions until soft and translucent.
2. Now, put in the sausage and cook an additional three minutes,

3. Mix in tomatoes, broth, water, sea salt, black pepper, crushed chili, and Italian seasonings.

4. Secure the lid. Choose "Manual" mode and High pressure; cook for five minutes. Once cooking is complete, use a quick pressure release; cautiously remove the lid.

5. Top with shaved Parmigiano-Reggiano cheese and serve warm

Nutritional Info: 340 Calories ‖ 27.9g Fat ‖ 5g Total Carbs ‖ 14.1g Protein ‖ 2.6g Sugars

Italian Summer Squash Soup

Time To Prepare: ten minutes
Time to Cook: fifteen minutes
Yield: Servings 4

Ingredients:

- ½ cup shredded carrot
- 1 cup shredded yellow squash
- 1 cup shredded zucchini
- 1 garlic clove, minced
- 1 small red onion, thinly cut
- 1 tablespoon finely chopped fresh chives
- 1 teaspoon salt
- 2 tablespoons finely chopped fresh basil
- 2 tablespoons pine nuts
- 3 cups vegetable broth
- 3 tablespoons extra-virgin olive oil

Directions:

1. In a large pot, heat the oil using high heat.
2. Put in the onion and garlic and sauté until tender, five to seven minutes.

3. Put in the zucchini, yellow squash, and carrot and sauté until tender, one to two minutes.

4. Pour the broth and salt then bring to its boiling point.

5. Reduce the heat and cook until the vegetables are soft, one to two minutes.

6. Mix in the basil and chives and serve, sprinkled with the pine nuts.

Nutritional Info: Calories: 172 ‖ Total Fat: 15g ‖ Total Carbohydrates: 6g ‖ Sugar: 3g ‖ Fiber: 2g ‖ Protein: 5g ‖ Sodium: 1170mg

Kumara & Chickpea Soup

Time To Prepare: twenty-five minutes
Time to Cook: thirty-five minutes
Yield: Servings 6

Ingredients:

- 1 bay leaf
- 1 onion (chopped)
- 1 teaspoon dried basil
- 1 tomato (chopped)
- ½ teaspoon dried thyme
- 1/4 teaspoon paprika
- 2 cloves garlic (minced)
- 2 cups kumara (peeled, chopped)
- 2 tablespoons olive oil
- 200g garbanzo beans
- 3 cups chicken broth
- Ground black pepper
- Mixed vegetables
- Salt

Directions:

1. Sauté onion, garlic, and sweet potatoes in oil for five minutes.

2. Put in broth, bay leaf, herbs, and seasoning.
3. Boil until soft.
4. Put in tomato, beans, and chickpeas, simmering some more before you serve.

Nutritional Info: Calories: 197 kcal ‖ Carbohydrates: 30 g ‖ Fat: 6 g ‖ Protein: 7.5 g

Lamb Stew

Time To Prepare: five minutes

Time to Cook: 8 hours

Yield: Servings 6

Ingredients:

- 1 lamb stock cube
- 1 onion, roughly chopped
- 2 pounds (907 g) boneless lamb, cut into cubes
- 2 tablespoons olive oil, plus more for greasing the frying pan
- 2 teaspoons dried rosemary
- 3 cups water
- 4 garlic cloves, finely chopped
- From the cupboard:
- Salt and freshly ground black pepper, to taste

Directions:

1. Position the lamb into a mildly greased nonstick frying pan, and cook using high heat for a couple of minutes or until browned.

2. Grease a slow cooker with olive oil, then put in the cooked lamb, stock cube, rosemary, onion, garlic, salt, black pepper, and 3 cups of water. Blend to blend well.

3. Place the slow cooker lid on and cook on LOW for eight hours.

4. Take away the cooked lamb stew from the slow cooker and serve warm.

Nutritional Info: calories: 252 ‖ total fat: 9.5g ‖ carbs: 4.9g ‖ protein: 34.9g

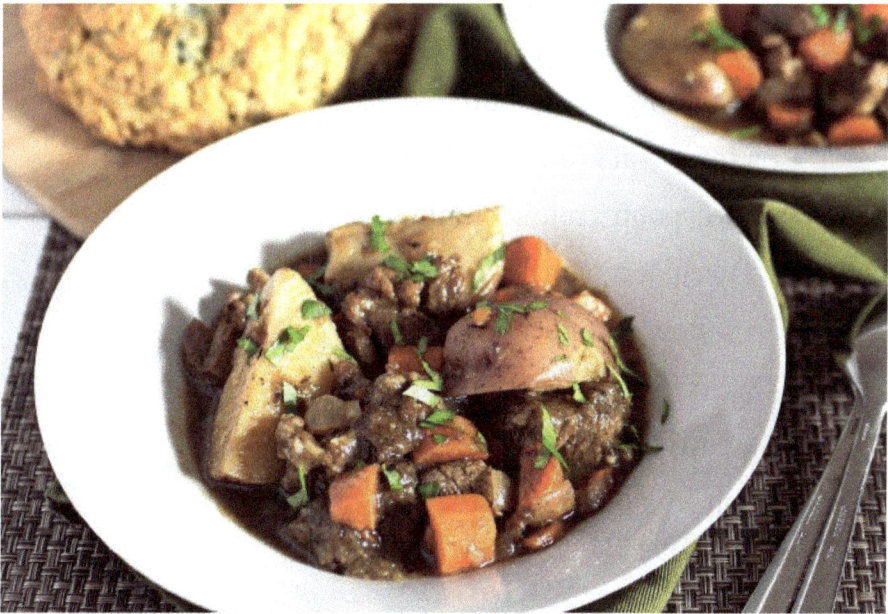

Lamb Taco Soup

Time To Prepare: ten minutes

Time to Cook: 4-6 hours minutes

Yield: Servings 6

Ingredients:

- ½ teaspoon cayenne pepper
- 1 cup diced tomatoes
- 1 cup shredded cheddar cheese
- 1 green bell pepper, chopped
- 1 pound ground lamb
- 1 teaspoon ground coriander
- 1 teaspoon ground cumin
- 1 teaspoon paprika
- 1 yellow onion, chopped
- 2 cloves garlic, chopped
- 4 cups beef broth
- Salt & pepper, to taste

Directions:

1. Put in all the ingredients to a slow cooker minus the shredded cheese and cook on high for four to 6 hours.
2. Mix in the shredded cheese before you serve.

Nutritional Info: Calories: 265 ‖ Carbohydrates: 6g ‖ Fiber: 1g Net ‖ Carbohydrates: 5g ‖ Fat: 13g ‖ Protein: 30g

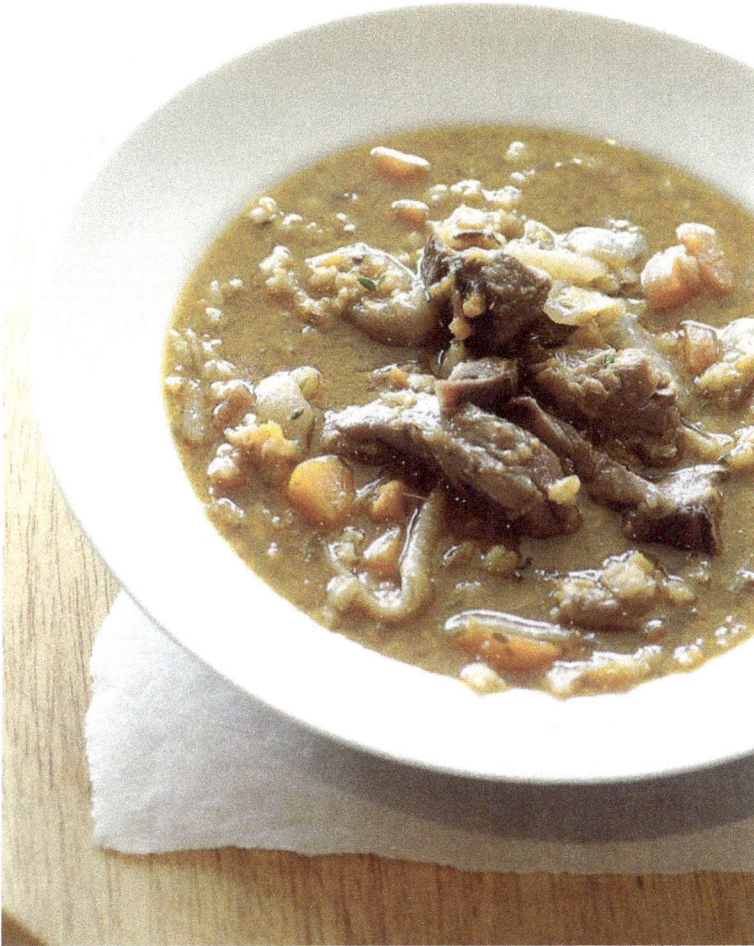

Lebanese Lentil Soup

Time To Prepare: fifteen minutes

Time to Cook: 60 minutes

Yield: Servings 6

Ingredients:

- 1 cup brown lentils
- 1 lemon juiced
- 1 medium onion
- 1 tablespoon olive oil
- 2 medium carrots
- 2 teaspoons cinnamon
- 2 teaspoons cumin
- 3 stalks celery
- 4 cloves garlic
- 4 cups chicken broth low sodium
- 4 cups water
- 8 cups spinach
- salt& pepper to taste

Directions:

1. Over moderate heat, heat oil in a soup pot, Put in & cook carrots, celery & onions until become soft for seven minutes, put in pepper & salt to taste.

2. Stir cumin, cinnamon & garlic heat it for 30-60 minutes. Put in lentils & heat for a couple of minutes to slightly toast. Pour in the lemon juice, water & chicken broth, then bring the pot to its boiling point. When lentils are soft, decrease the heat to low & simmer, approximately 30-45 minutes.

3. Before you serve, mix in the spinach, cook until the color is green, now served to put in pepper, lemon juice & salt.

Nutritional Info: Calories: 102 kcal ‖ Protein: 6.33 g ‖ Fat: 4.58 g ‖ Carbohydrates: 11.6 g

Leek, Chicken and Spinach Soup

Time To Prepare: ten minutes
Time to Cook: fifteen minutes
Yield: Servings 4

Ingredients:

- ¼ teaspoon freshly ground black pepper
- 1 tablespoon thinly cut fresh chives
- 1 teaspoon salt
- 2 cups shredded rotisserie chicken
- 2 leeks, white parts only, thinly cut
- 2 teaspoons grated or minced lemon zest
- 3 tablespoons unsalted butter
- 4 cups baby spinach
- 4 cups chicken broth

Directions:

1. In a large pot, melt the butter on high heat.
2. Put in the leeks and sauté until tender and starting to brown, three to five minutes.
3. Put in the spinach, broth, salt, and pepper and bring to its boiling point.

4. Reduce the heat and cook till the spinach wilts, one to two minutes.

5. Place the chicken and cook until warmed through one to two minutes.

6. Drizzle with the chives and lemon zest before you serve.

Nutritional Info: Calories: 256 ‖ Total Fat: 12g ‖ Total Carbohydrates: 9g ‖ Sugar: 3g ‖ Fiber: 2g ‖ Protein: 27g ‖ Sodium: 1483mg

DESSERTS

Fruit Salad

Time To Prepare: 10 Minutes

Time to Cook: 20 Minutes

Yield: Servings 2-3

Ingredients:

- ½ of 1 Watermelon, chopped into little pieces
- 1 Pineapple, cut into little pieces
- 1 Pomegranate, small
- 1 Red Papaya, cut into little pieces
- 1 tsp. Ginger, freshly grated
- 4 Strawberries, chopped
- Dash of Turmeric

Directions:

1. To start with, place all the fruits in a large-sized container.
2. Next, spoon in the turmeric and ginger over the fruits.
3. Toss thoroughly before you serve.

Nutritional Info: ‖ Calories: 118Kcal ‖ Protein: 1.6g ‖ Carbohydrates: 36.6g ‖ Fat: 0.5g

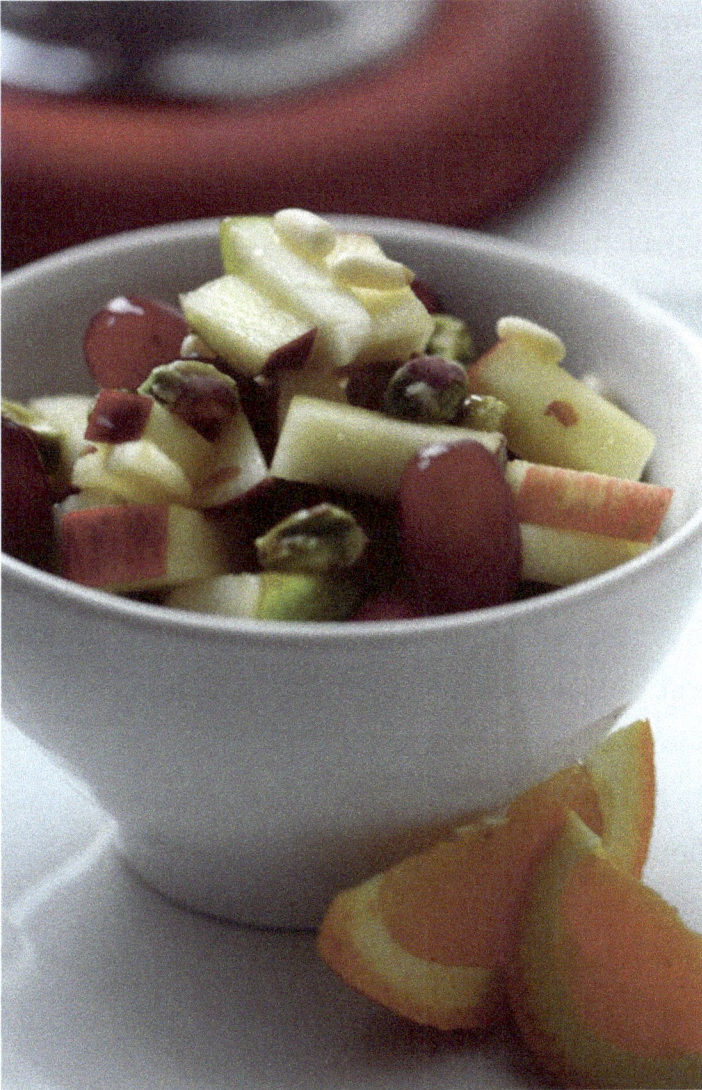

Glazed Banana

Time To Prepare: ten minutes

Time to Cook: five minutes

Yield: Servings 2

Ingredients:

- 1 peeled and cut under-ripened banana
- 1 tbsp. of filtered water
- 1 tbsp. of olive oil
- 1 tbsp. of raw honey
- 1/8 tsp. of ground cinnamon

Directions:

1. In a nonstick frying pan, warm oil on moderate heat.
2. Put in banana slices and cook for approximately 1-2 minutes per side.
3. In the meantime, in a small container, put in water and honey and beat thoroughly.
4. Move the banana slices on a serving plate.
5. Instantly, pour honey mixture over banana slices.
6. Keep aside to cool to room temperature. Serve with the drizzling of cinnamon.

Nutritional Info: ‖ Calories: 145 ‖ Fat: 7.2g ‖ Carbohydrates: 22.2g ‖ Protein: 0.7g ‖ Fiber: 1.6g

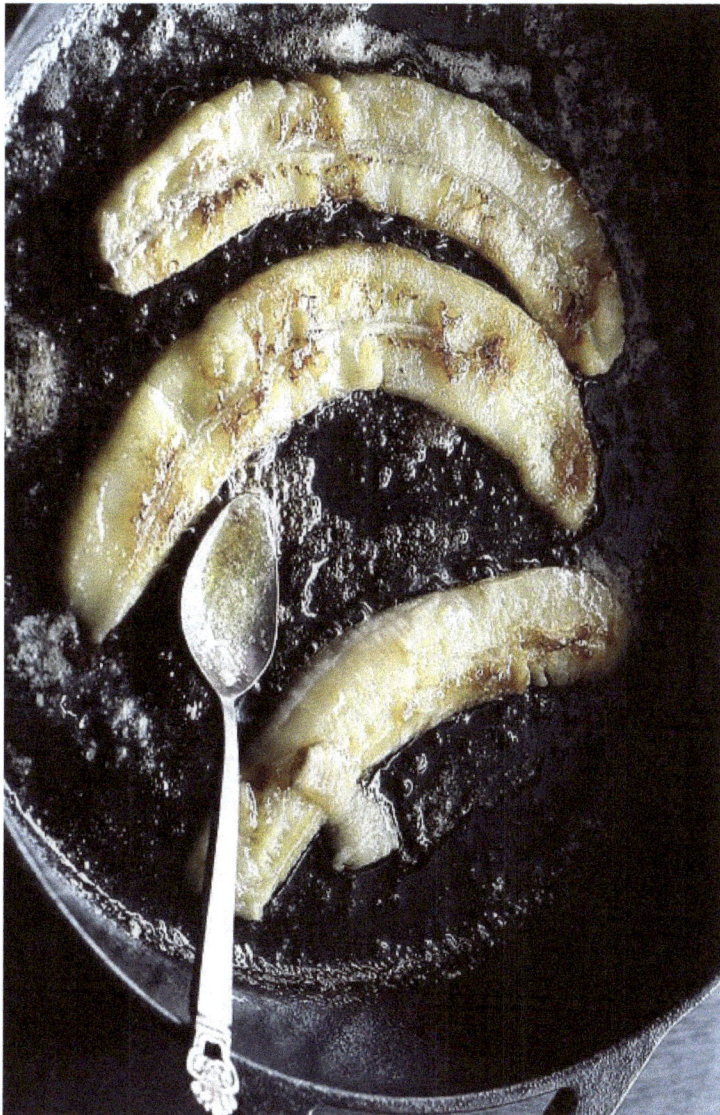

Glorious Blueberry Crumble

Time To Prepare: ten minutes

Time to Cook: thirty minutes

Yield: Servings 6

Ingredients:

- ½ cup of softened coconut oil
- ½ tsp. of ground cinnamon
- 1 cup of almond meal
- 1 cup of toasted and finely crushed almonds
- 2 tbsp. of coconut sugar
- 4 cups of fresh blueberries

Directions:

1. Set the oven to 350F then lightly, grease a pie dish.
2. In a huge container, combine all ingredients apart from blueberries.
3. Split half of the almond mixture at the bottom of the prepared pie dish.
4. Put blueberries over almond mixture uniformly.
5. Top with the rest of the almond mixture uniformly.
6. Bake for minimum 30 minutes or till the top becomes golden brown.
7. Serve warm.

Nutritional Info: ‖ Calories: 411 ‖ Fat: 34.3g ‖ Carbohydrates: 24.9g ‖ Protein: 7.4g ‖ Fiber: 6.4g

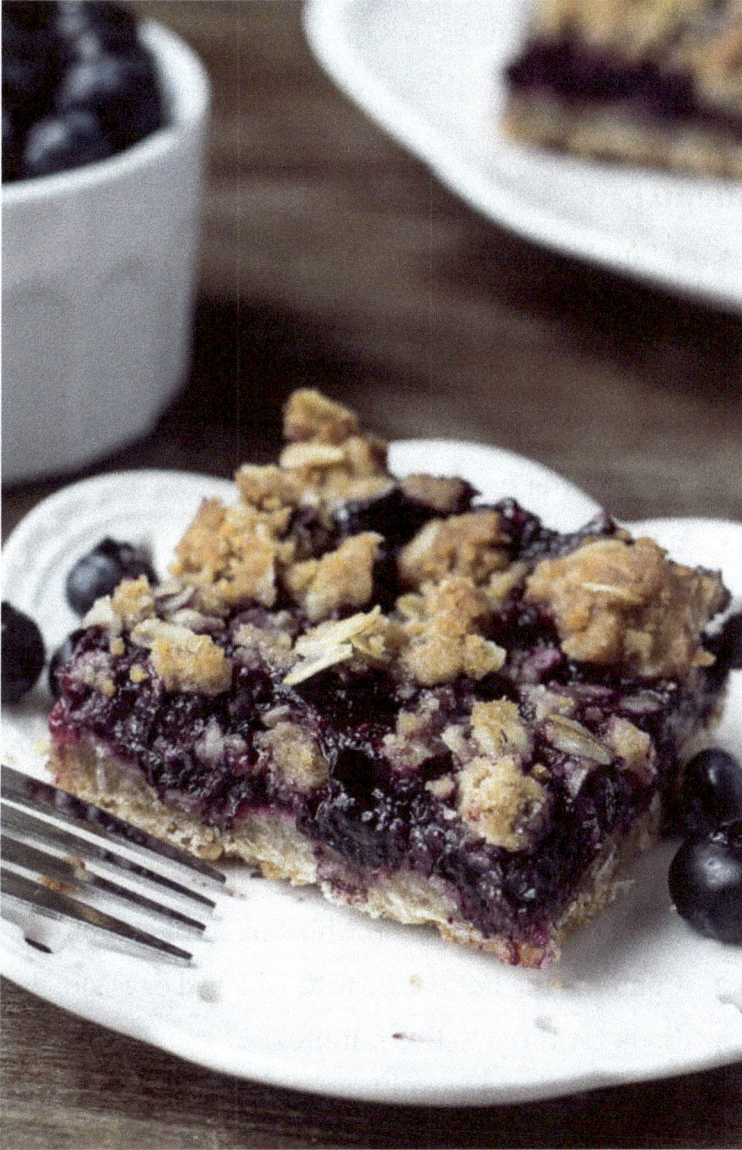

Green Tea Pudding

Time To Prepare: twenty minutes

Time to Cook: ten minutes

Yield: Servings 3

Ingredients:

- 1 Tsp. Matcha Green Tea Powder
- 1/4 Cup Brown Sugar
- 1/4 Cup Corn Starch
- 1/8-Tbsp. Cinnamon Powder
- 100g Butter
- 2 Cup Heavy Milk
- 3 Eggs
- Salt

Directions:

1. In a big pot, mix brown sugar, milk, cornstarch, and matcha powder.
2. In moderate heat, keep whisking until combined.
3. Combine the hot batter with whisked eggs slowly.
4. Cook for three to five minutes.
5. Strain the mixture and put in butter.
6. Place the mixture in a container, place in your fridge for a few hours before you serve.

Nutritional Info: ‖ Calories: 359 kcal ‖ Carbohydrates: 60 g ‖ Fat: 3.0 g ‖ Protein: 18.4 g

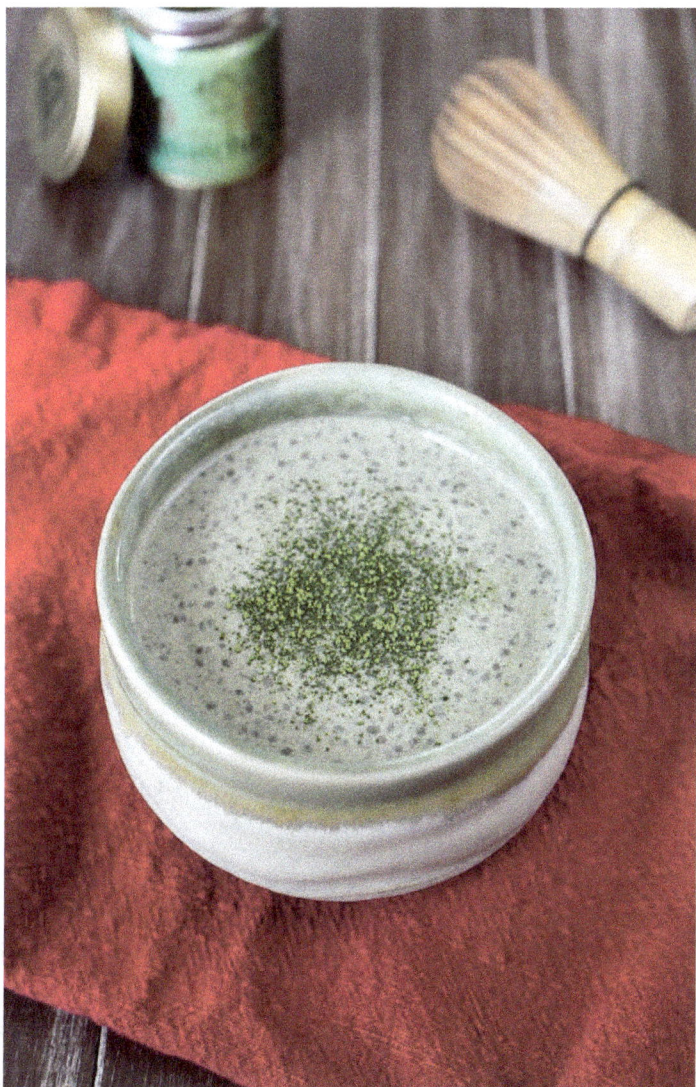

Grilled Peaches

Time To Prepare: ten minutes

Time to Cook: ten minutes

Yield: Servings 6

Ingredients:

- ¼ cup of walnuts, chopped
- ½ cup of coconut cream
- 1 teaspoon of organic vanilla extract
- 3 medium peaches (halved and pitted)
- Ground cinnamon

Directions:

1. Preheat the grill on moderate to low heat. Grease the grill grate.
2. Position the peach slices on the grill with the cut-side down.
3. Grill each side for three to five minutes or until the desired doneness is attained.
4. .In the meantime, mix coconut cream with vanilla extract in a container. Beat until the desired smoothness is achieved.
5. Ladle the whipped cream over each peach half.
6. Top with walnuts and drizzle with cinnamon. Serve instantly.

Nutritional Info: ‖ Calories: 110 ‖ Fat: 8g ‖ Carbohydrates: 8.8g ‖ Sugar: 7.8g ‖ Protein: 2.4g ‖ Sodium: 3mg

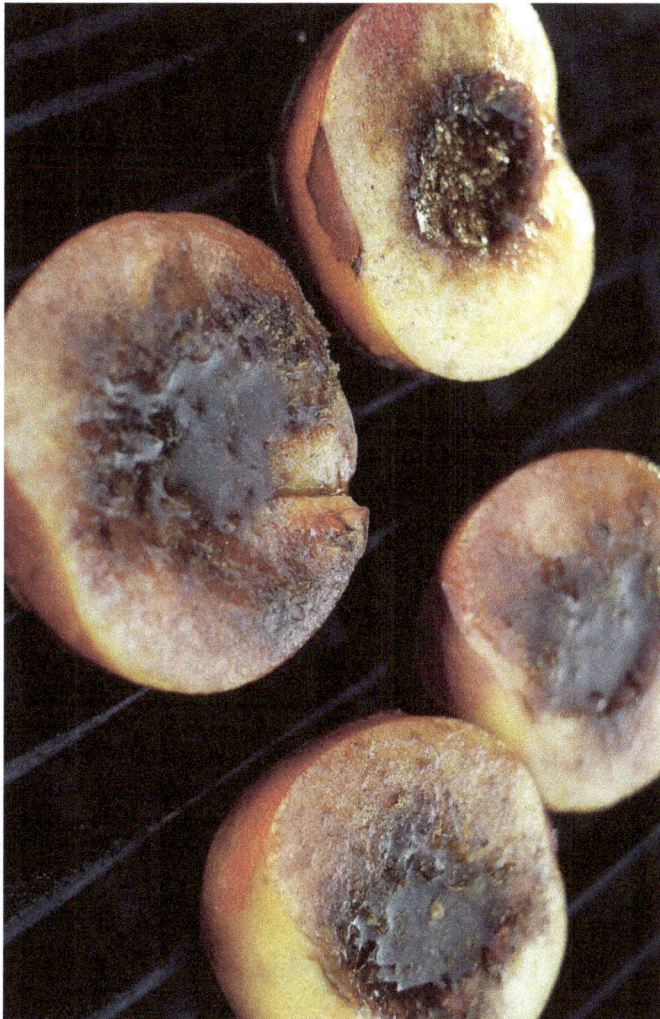

Hot Chocolate

Time To Prepare: 5 Minutes
Time to Cook: 5 Minutes
Yield: Servings 2

Ingredients:

- ¼ tsp. Turmeric
- ½ tsp. Cinnamon
- 1 tbsp. Coconut Oil
- 1 tbsp. Honey, raw
- 2 cups Almond Milk
- 2 tbsp. Cocoa Powder, unsweetened

Directions:

1. To start with, bring the almond milk to its boiling point in a deep deep cooking pan on moderate heat.
2. Now, bring this mixture to a simmer and then mix in the cocoa powder to it.
3. Next, spoon in the turmeric powder and cinnamon to it. Mix thoroughly/
4. Next, put in honey to it and once blended well, put in the coconut oil
5. Give the drink a good stir until everything comes together.

6. Serve instantly.

Nutritional Info: ‖ Calories: 150 Kcal ‖ Protein: 2.1g ‖ Carbohydrates: 15.2g ‖ Fat: 11.1gm

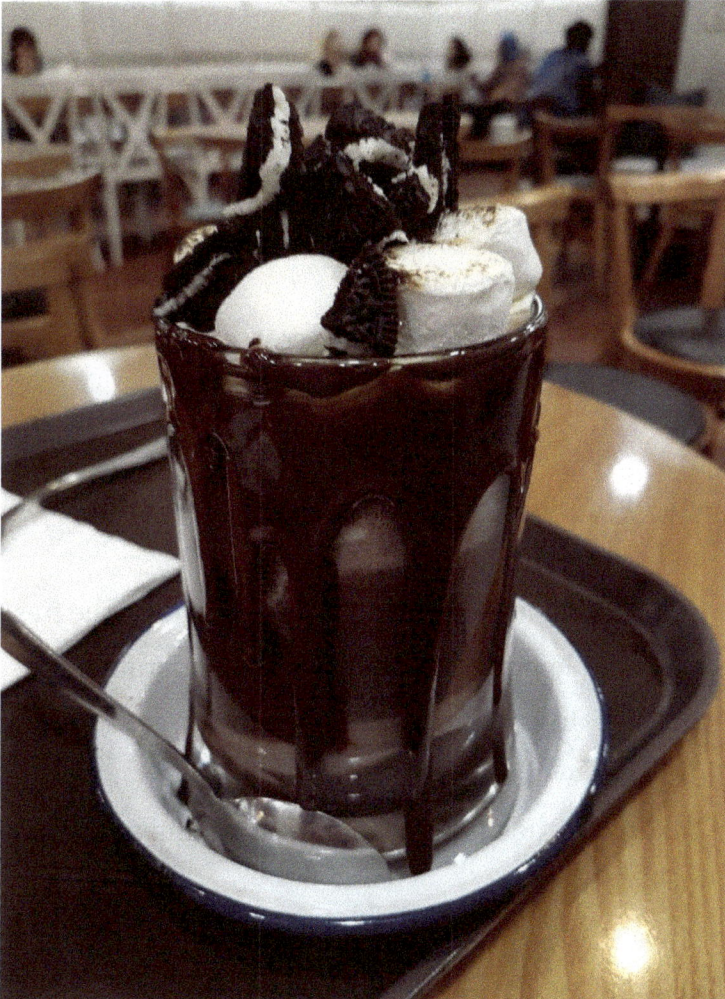

Lemon Sorbet

Time To Prepare: ten minutes

Time to Cook: 0 minutes

Yield: Servings 2

Ingredients:

- ½ cup of raw honey
- ½ cups of fresh lemon juice
- 2 cups of filtered water
- 2 tablespoons of fresh lemon zest, grated

Directions:

1. Put into your freezer the ice-cream maker tub for a day before making the sorbet.
2. Combine all ingredients in a pan, excluding the freshly squeezed lemon juice and cook on moderate heat.
3. Simmer for minimum 1 minute, up to the sugar dissolves while stirring constantly.
4. Take away the mixture from the heat and put in lemon juice.
5. Move the combination to an airtight container and place in your fridge for around 2hours.
6. Put it into an ice-cream maker and process according to the manufacturer's instructions.

7. Put in one tablespoon of oil when the motor is running.
8. Return the ice-cream into the airtight container and freeze for roughly 2 hours.

Nutritional Info: ‖ Calories: 305 ‖ Fat: 1.5g ‖ Carbohydrates: 74.9g ‖ Sugar: 73.8g ‖ Protein: 1.9g ‖ Sodium: 40mg

Lemon Vegan Cake

Time To Prepare: ten minutes

Time to Cook: ten minutes

Yield: Servings 3

Ingredients:

- ½ lemon extract
- 1 cup of pitted dates
- 1 lemon juice and zest
- 1½ cup agave
- 1½ cups of dairy-free yogurt
- 1½ cups pineapple, crushed
- 1½ teaspoon vanilla extract
- 2½ cups pecans ½
- 3 avocados, halved & pitted
- 3 cups of cauliflower rice, prepared
- Pinch of cinnamon

Directions:

1. Coat your baking sheet using parchment paper.
2. Pulse the pecans in a food processor.
3. Put in the agave and dates. Pulse for one minute.

4. Move this mix to the baking sheet. Wipe the container of your processor.

5. Combine the pineapple, agave, avocados, cauliflower, lemon juice, and zest in a food processor. Pulse till smooth

6. Now put in the lemon extract, cinnamon, and vanilla extract. Pulse.

7. Pour this mix into your pan, on the crust.

8. Place in your fridge for around five hours at least.

9. Take out the cake and keep it at room temperature for about twenty minutes.

10. Take out the cake's outer ring.

11. Mix together the vanilla extract, agave, and yogurt in a container.

12. Pour on your cake.

Nutritional Info: Calories 688 ‖ Carbohydrates: 100g ‖ Fat: 28g ‖ Protein: 9g ‖ Sugar: 40g

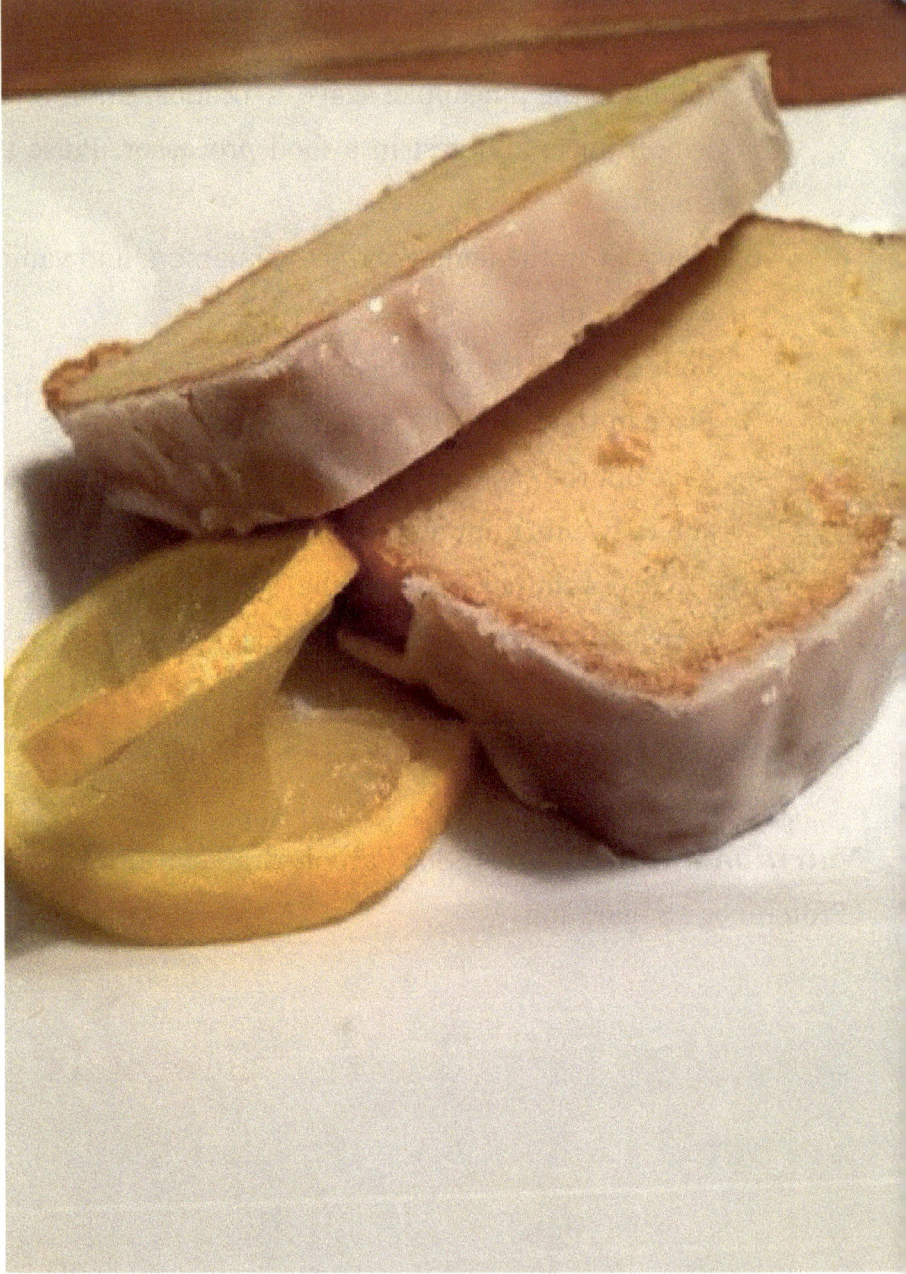

Lemonade Ice Pops

Time To Prepare: 4 hours and ten minutes

Time to Cook: 0 minutes

Yield: Servings 4

Ingredients:

- 1 cup hot water
- 2 cups cold water
- 2 iced tea and lemonade tea bags

Directions:

1. Put hot water in a container, put in tea bags, cover, and set aside for about ten minutes to steep. Squeeze the tea bags to take off all the water and then discard them. Put in cold water, split into your ice pop maker, freeze for around six hours, before you serve.

2. Enjoy!

Nutritional Info: ‖ Calories: 38 ‖ Fat: 0 ‖ Fiber: 0 ‖ Carbohydrates: 0 ‖ Protein: 1

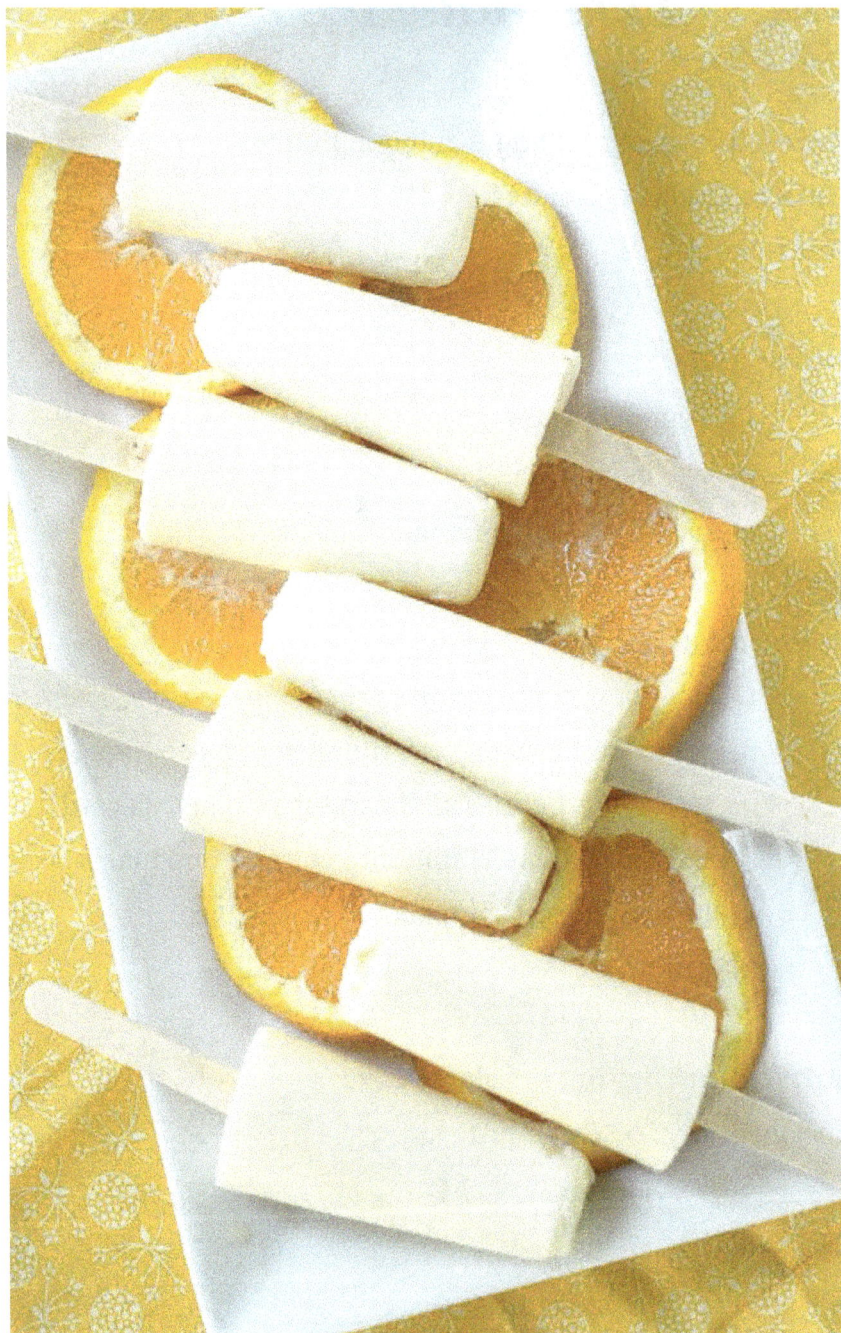

Matcha and Blueberries Pudding

Time To Prepare: three hours

Time to Cook: 0 minutes

Yield: Servings 2

Ingredients:

- 1 banana, cut
- 1 cup blueberries
- 1 cup matcha green tea powder
- 2 cups almond milk
- 4 tablespoons chia seeds

Directions:

1. Put chia seeds, milk and matcha powder in a container. Stir, cover, then place in your fridge for around three hours. Split into bowls, top with banana slices and blueberries before you serve.
2. Enjoy!

Nutritional Info: ‖ Calories: 324 ‖ Fat: 9 ‖ Fiber: 18 ‖ Carbohydrates: 24 ‖ Protein: 8

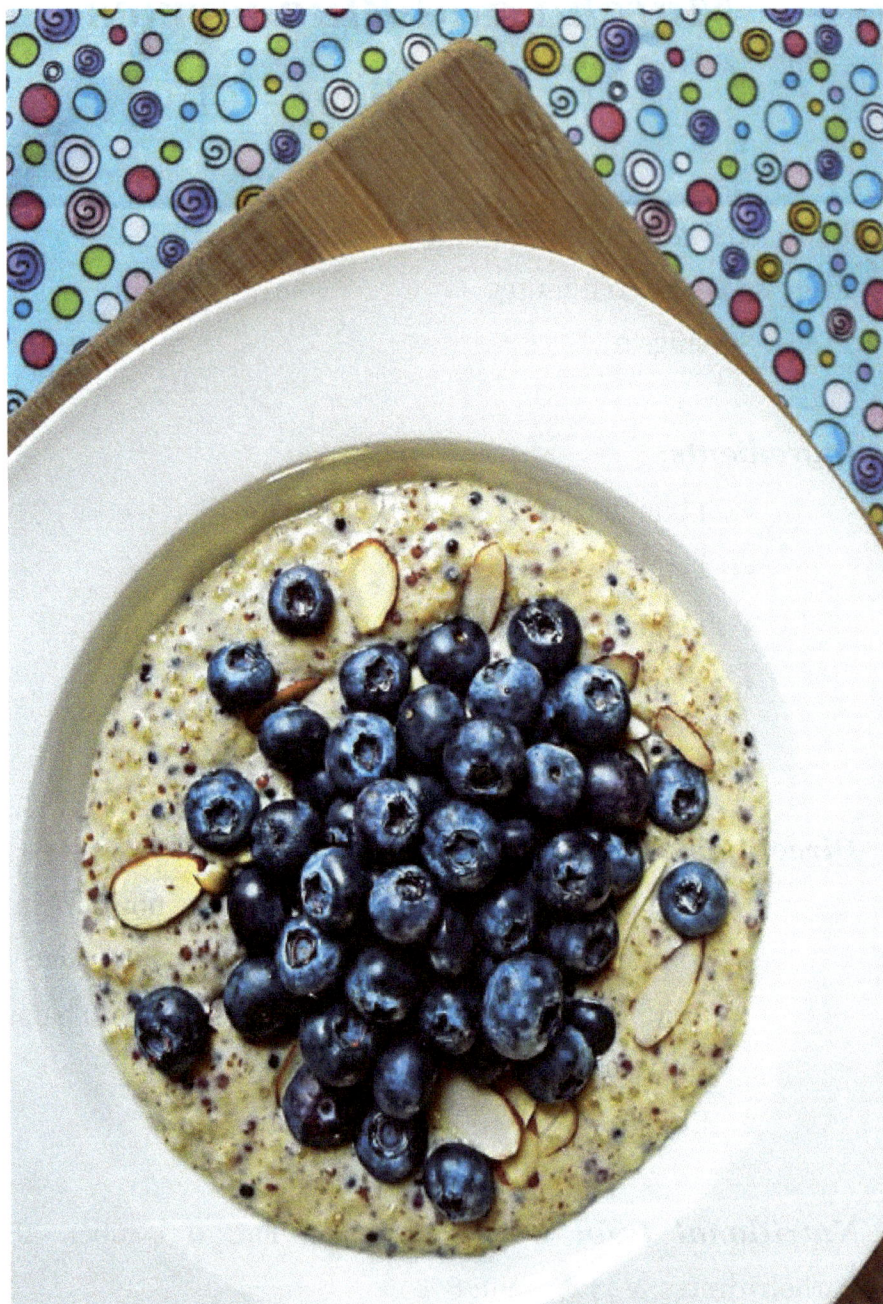

www.ingramcontent.com/pod-product-compliance
Lightning Source LLC
Chambersburg PA
CBHW070735030426
42336CB00013B/1979